Care of the
SICK CHILD

Jane Coffey

Hodder & Stoughton

A MEMBER OF THE HODDER HEADLINE GROUP

British Library Cataloguing in Publication Data

A catalogue for this title is available from the British Library.

ISBN 0 340 61018 2

First published 1995
Impression number 10 9 8 7 6 5 4 3 2 1
Year   1999 1998 1997 1996 1995

Typeset by Wearset, Boldon, Tyne and Wear.
Printed in Great Britain for Hodder & Stoughton Educational, a division of Hodder Headline Plc, 338 Euston Road, London NW1 3BH by Page Brothers, Norwich, Norfolk.

CONTENTS

INTRODUCTION

In recent years, I have been involved with the Business Technical Education Council (BTEC) National Diploma and Certificate in Caring (Nursery Nursing) and National Vocational Qualification courses and have been surprised to find that there are few books written for course units at these levels.

I was particularly surprised, when I started teaching Care of the Sick Child, at the lack of suitable material. There are plenty of excellent books written for parents on caring of ill children, but they do not meet the specialist requirements of the courses. There are plenty of excellent paediatric books written for nurses; however, much of the material is too detailed.

Caring for children is one of the most fulfilling and rewarding occupations anyone can have. It is a great privilege to look after other people's children, but it lays a heavy responsibility on the carer to be competent in the recognition of illness and subsequent management of an ill child. This book has been written to provide the information necessary for a carer to meet these important needs.

Generally, ill children are much better off being cared for in their own homes by the most important carers of all – their parents. However children do become unwell at 'inconvenient' times of the day and, if they do, they deserve the very best care possible. In order for the carer to be able to provide that, he or she needs to have some understanding of the process of the illness and how to look after the child.

Carers working with children, whatever course they have completed or are in the process of completing, should find this book useful.

HOW TO USE THIS BOOK

—

This information is divided into meaningful sections, beginning with a general look at health and moving on to specific illnesses and care.

Some chapters are much longer than others, particularly those on infections and congenital abnormalities. However you are not expected to read all of this in one go; read the introduction and then turn to the relevant information as and when you need it.

This book does not set out to include first aid, although the author recommends that anyone caring for children should hold a first-aid certificate.

ACKNOWLEDGMENTS

—

I would like to thank my husband, Paul, for all the help, support and technical guidance he has given over the last few months – without him, I would certainly have given up. His contribution has been tremendously helpful. I would also like to thank my children, Laura, Patrick and Duncan, for their patience and encouragement which helped me to fulfil my ambition to write this book.

Thanks also to Frances Davies (Health Visitor, Oxfordshire Community Health NHS Trust) who very kindly took on the task of reading (and re-reading) the script and making helpful suggestions. She has taught me such a lot, and I am extremely grateful to her.

To Aidan MacFarlane (Consultant Community Paediatrician) for general encouragement and advice, particularly on the *Failure to Thrive* section, and to Tam Fry (Child Growth Foundation) for his advice and for providing the new growth charts included in this book. I am also very grateful to Denis Lawlor, who has patiently helped me to cope with the intricacies of word processing, which I found almost more daunting than writing the book.

FACTORS INFLUENCING CHILD HEALTH

—

•A century ago six babies out of ten survived to adulthood, such were the ravages of disease, undernourishment, squalor and ignorance.•
Prevention and health: everybody's business

In 1948 the World Health Organisation defined health as 'a state of complete physical, mental and social well-being, not merely the absence of disease or infirmity . . .'

Usually, it is the family which provides the environment to meet the physical, mental and social needs of a child so that he or she is offered emotional security.

The health of a child is influenced by many factors. These may be considered as belonging to two main groups. The first is the physical make-up of the child, which usually cannot be affected to any great extent after birth. This includes inherited conditions and the effect of intra-uterine conditions, such as nutrition and smoking.

The second is the effect of the child's environment, which may, of course, be influenced and altered. The environment is the home and family and the larger outside world, which includes the country, its culture, its levels of air, water and land pollution and other variables.

Some Influences on Child Health this Century

These comments on this century's influences on health care are by no means exhaustive; the aim is simply to set the scene for the rest of the book and hopefully to stimulate interest in the major influences on child health.

HEALTH CARE AND THE NATIONAL HEALTH SERVICE

The National Health Service came into effect in 1948. It provided health care paid for by the tax payer, and was therefore free when required. It was designed to be available regardless of social status or ability to pay. However, the Black Report (1984) suggests that there are still inequalities in health related to social status, although these are clearly much less than prior to 1948.

The National Health Service provides care for mothers and children via Primary and Secondary Health Care.

Primary Health Care

The Primary Health Care team is made up of a multi-disciplinary team of personnel, including general practitioners, practice nurses (those that work in the health centre or medical centre), community nurses (those that work in the district), health visitors and community midwives. Some Primary Health Care teams include the social worker, the school nurse and the community psychiatric nurse. The team is supported by receptionists and secretaries. This team caters for the medical, nursing and social work needs of the community, and individuals may be based in the health centre or operate from separate areas, but they will usually meet regularly to discuss issues. Many clinics are provided via this service, including antenatal clinics, child surveillance clinics (this is covered in detail in the next chapter) and the school health service.

Secondary Health Care

The country is divided into areas, and each area has its own District Hospital, which provides the services not offered by the Primary Health Care team.

ANTENATAL CARE

This is a good example of care which may be offered either by the Primary Health Care team or by the Hospital Service, or which can be shared between the two.

All mothers are offered free antenatal care. The aims of this care are to:

• promote a safe and healthy pregnancy and a safe delivery for both mother and baby;

- prevent avoidable complications by identifying any deviation from the norm and minimise the effects of any unavoidable complications;
- screen for conditions that may have an adverse effect on the mother or baby;
- prepare for labour and parenthood.

Antenatal care has had a direct effect on the reduction of infant mortality and maternal mortality rates this century.

PREVENTION OF INFECTION

In the past, infection was a major cause of mortality and morbidity in Britain. During this century, deaths from infectious diseases have been dramatically reduced. However, immunisation was not the sole reason for this; other factors also had an effect:

- better housing and thus less overcrowding;
- improved sanitation and water supplies leading to improved hygiene;
- improved nutrition;
- antibiotics from the 1940s;
- health education;
- changes in the virulence of some micro-organisms.

In 1990, the Government set the National Target level for immunisations at ninety per cent of all children. Immunisations are generally carried out wherever the child attends the child surveillance clinic. In 1995, it is likely that this will be increased to ninety-five per cent. It is important to maintain a high rate of immunisation, and therefore immunity, so that the incidence of disease may be kept low.

SPECIAL-CARE BABY UNITS

These are found in maternity units in many hospitals. Babies with problems at birth can be cared for by specially trained staff using sophisticated equipment in these units. This has resulted in premature babies having an increased chance of survival.

CONTRACEPTION

Prior to 1921, when Dr Marie Stopes opened the first family planning clinic (birth control clinic), there was no formal contraception service. From 1967, these clinics were able to provide birth control on social as well as medical grounds. The effect of planned pregnancies has a positive influence on child health. In recent years, advice on contraception has often been given by the Primary Health Care team, and many of the family planning clinics have closed.

NUTRITION

The nutritional status of children in Britain has improved over the last century. However, specialist advice may be necessary from dieticians, both in the community and in hospitals.

Pregnant mothers are given the opportunity to discuss the positive effects of breast feeding, both at the antenatal and the child surveillance clinic. This initiative was introduced in response to a move away from breast feeding when formulated baby milks became available. The child surveillance clinic also offers advice and support on many aspects of nutrition, including the recommendations for giving vitamin drops to all children from the age of six months to two years and preferably to five years. Fluoride supplements are recommended for children in areas where there are insufficient quantities in the water supply. This clinic also gives advice on many financial benefits to which the mother and child may be entitled.

Some education authorities offer free milk (⅓ pint per day) to children in play groups or nursery schools. Some also offer free school meals to economically disadvantaged children, and in general a school meals service has improved the diet of many children, although it is no longer a statutory provision.

HOUSING

Health Care teams are concerned about housing, but control is not in their hands. Food, shelter and warmth are basic needs, all of which are provided in the home. Poor housing and overcrowding can have a profound effect on the physical, mental, social and emotional well-being of the child (and parents).

ATMOSPHERIC EFFECTS

Health Care teams are concerned about the effect of the atmosphere on health.

There are a number of pollutants in air that are hazardous to health. These include chemicals, smoke, ozone and dust. The Clean Air act was introduced in 1956 to reduce the pollution in the cities, but air pollution is on the increase again. Ingestion of lead is associated with a number of health problems, such as behavioural difficulties and underachievement. To reduce the risks, all cars built since 1991 run on lead-free petrol.

Epidemiology

Epidemiology is the study of factors affecting disease in a given population. It is important to study such factors, because information gathered on aspects of child health assist in planning health care provision, preventing illness and controlling the spread of illness.

Epidemiologists study groups of individuals (populations) to investigate the numbers affected by an aspect of health. Information needs to be collected from a cross-section of people, both healthy and sick, in order to determine the numbers of ill people in a given population. This information may be collected nationally or locally, depending on the nature of the study. It can, for instance, be collected routinely from registration of births and deaths, or the information can be collected by the population census every ten years or by specific surveys set up to study a specific population or disease, as in the Black Report (1984) referred to earlier. Information is published yearly via the Office of Population Censuses and Surveys (OPCS), including information on the social class of those surveyed, their age and causes of death.

PUBLISHED STATISTICS

The information collected annually by the OPCS is divided into information on mortality and morbidity.

Mortality

This is information gathered on numbers and causes of death. Infant and perinatal mortality rates are indicators of the health status of a population.

Infant mortality rate
This is the number of deaths of infants under the age of one year per 1000 live births.

Note: the infant mortality rate of children born into families of social class V (unskilled workers) is twice that of children born to social class I (professional families).

Perinatal mortality rate
This is the number of stillbirths (death of the foetus after the twenty-eighth week of pregnancy) and deaths that occur within the first week of life.

Note: the perinatal mortality rate of children born to social class V (unskilled workers) is more than three times greater than children born to social class I (professional families).

Neonatal mortality rate
The number of deaths within the first four weeks of life. The common causes of death during this period are related to immaturity, congenital abnormalities and infections.

Maternal mortality rate
The number of deaths of women associated with childbirth per 1000 births. Maternal mortality rates have fallen since 1935.

Morbidity

This is information on illness, whether caused by disease, injury or disability. However, it is more difficult to collect information on morbidity, because the collection relies on reports from many sources, and not all cases are reported. Morbidity is measured as **prevalence** (the proportion of a group of people having a condition at any one time) and **incidence** (the number of new cases reported within a stated time).

Information can be collected via the census and through notification of certain infectious diseases which have to be reported. General practitioners, hospitals and social security departments keep various registers which provide information for the surveys, such as the child protection register.

With increasing computerisation, information gathering should become easier and more reliable.

STUDENT ACTIVITIES

Antenatal Care

1   It might be possible, after consulting with a course tutor and gaining permission from the health care professionals involved, to visit an antenatal clinic to observe how these aims are met. Remember that the carer must be aware of the need for confidentiality.

Prevention of Infection

1   Familiarise yourself with the immunisation schedules currently recommended in the UK. What advice is the parent given after the child has been immunised?

2   Consider each of the factors from the text (i.e. better housing and therefore less overcrowding, improved sanitation and water supplies leading to improved hygiene, improved nutrition, antibiotic from 1940s, health education and changes in the virulence of some micro-organism) and write notes on how you think each factor might have an effect on the reduction of deaths from infectious diseases. Give examples wherever possible.

Nutrition

1   You are working as a nursery nurse alongside the health visitor. You have been asked to give a fifteen-minute talk to a group of eight parents at a parentcraft class on the importance of giving fluoride supplements to children and its positive effect on teeth. Outline the forms you think this session might take. Consider the following: How you might most effectively get the information across? What visual aids will you use? It is often a good idea to give the parent(s) some information to take away for consideration. The health education department may have several leaflets on the subject – look at them and find out which ones might be the best to use. Find out the fluoride levels in your water supply and whether supplements are recommended for children.

Housing

There are large numbers of homeless families in Britain today. Discuss with colleagues how this may affect the health and well-being of children. *A Bad Start in Life – Children, Health and Housing* by Annette Furley, published by Shelter publications, is a good reference.

Atmospheric Effects

1   There is an increased amount of traffic on Britain's roads. List the possible pollutants and give a brief description of the effects of each on children's health.

2   Direct and prolonged exposure to sunlight has been implicated as a cause of skin cancer. Design a poster to be put up in the child surveillance clinic showing how to protect a child against the hazards of sunlight.

Morbidity

Familiarise yourself with *Social Trends* (published by the Central Statistical Office), which gives information on health-related issues, and *Population Trends* (published by the Office of Population Censuses and Surveys), which gives information on the population and statistics on health. Both these publications can be found in most libraries.

2

CHILD HEALTH SURVEILLANCE

—

Mothers are invited to bring their children to the child health clinics at regular intervals during their pre-school years. The aims of the child health clinic are:

- to promote health and prevent illness;
- to allow early detection of any abnormalities and problems and therefore give early treatment.

The clinics achieve these aims by inviting babies and children to be seen at regular intervals; between six and eight weeks old, six and nine months old, two years and four and a half years.

The philosophy of the clinics is to welcome and encourage attendance, and they therefore tend to have a relaxed atmosphere. Toys are provided for the children, and they can mix with other children while their parent(s) talk to one another. In this way, the clinic encourages social interaction. This is an important spin-off, because many parents, particularly after the first baby, may feel lonely and isolated.

A health visitor may be present at the clinics and he or she will advise and give help as necessary; indeed, parents are often encouraged to drop in rather than attend only when the child has an appointment.

The friendly, welcoming approach helps put the parent at ease, and they are then happier to discuss any problems. Parents will be encouraged to talk to the doctor or health visitor about any worries.

Records

In recent years, a Personal Child Health Record has been produced, which allows the parents to keep a record of the child's development and progress. It is completed by doctors, health visitors and parents. The parents are encouraged to take this Personal Child Health Record everywhere with them. If the child is taken ill when the family is away for the weekend, or if the child is admitted to hospital, the Record will give the necessary information about the child.

STUDENT ACTIVITIES

Records

1   Familiarise yourself with the Personal Child Health Record book.

2   Ask permission from one of the health care professionals to observe a child health clinic and, ideally, health check on a child aged six to eight weeks, six to nine months, two years, and four and a half years. Remember that all observations must be treated in the strictest confidence. Keep a record of any new information you learn.

The Importance of Early Detection of Abnormalities

Early detection and treatment may improve a child's health by avoiding more serious consequences; for example, untreated congenital hip dislocation may lead to walking disability, which may ultimately lead to arthritis. Parents come to terms with an abnormality more easily if it is detected early and discussion and support is offered. Early detection may enable doctors to give advice on possible effects in subsequent pregnancies.

The Neonatal Examination

A **family history** is taken before the examination. This includes information on any medical conditions that might be transmitted to or affect the child in any way, for example a genetic condition, an infection, diabetes, hypertension, fits or any psychiatric illness.

A **social history** of the family is also taken. This includes the parents' employment status, housing, their smoking habits and alcohol intake.

All babies are examined as soon as possible after birth. The doctor will examine the baby in a methodical but opportunist way: for example, if the child is crying, the mouth can be examined at that time. Whilst the doctor is examining the baby, he or she will usually explain what he or she is doing and the reason for it. The nature of the examination is usually relaxed enough to allow for any questions and includes an examination of the following areas:

- physical development;
- motor system;
- manipulation;
- hearing and language;
- vision;
- social skills.

PHYSICAL DEVELOPMENT

Each of the following are noted and recorded.

- The **overall appearance** of the baby is examined. This may reveal abnormalities – low ears, a large bridge to the nose, slanted eyes – all of which may indicate a specific condition, such as Down's syndrome.
- The **weight** is noted on the centile chart (see page 69).
- The **head circumference** is measured and noted on the centile chart.
- The **fontanelles** (the soft spots on a baby's head where the skull is not fully formed) should be examined at this stage. Both the anterior and the posterior fontanelles should be felt (see figure 1). They should be soft to the touch and neither bulging nor dipping.

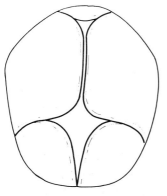

Posterior fontanelle (triangular shaped). Closes by two months, approximately.

Anterior fontanelle (diamond shaped). Closes by eighteen months, approximately.

Figure 1   Fontanelles

11

- The **mouth** is checked for the presence of a cleft palate (a small hole in the roof of the mouth (hard palate)). If present, this will need to be surgically repaired, since feeding may prove a problem. Sometimes a cleft palate is associated with a hare lip. This will be obvious to the doctor when he or she looks at the overall appearance of the baby, and the mother can be offered reassurance as this can be repaired surgically.
- The **skin** is checked for **colour**. The baby should be pink, but occasionally he or she will appear to have slightly blue hands and feet, particularly if examined very soon after birth; he or she usually 'pinks up' within a few minutes. A baby who appears to be blue around the mouth and lips will need urgent medical care, as this is an indication that the heart or lungs are not functioning properly. The **texture** of the skin will be noted. A premature baby may be covered with vernix (a greasy, protective covering over the skin). A post-term baby (born after 40 weeks' gestation) may be born with dry, flaky skin. **Pigmentation** is noted: for example, Mongolian blue spots (patches of darker pigmentation often found on the baby's back or buttocks that can be mistaken for bruises) are sometimes seen in children with black skin. Some children are born with **birth marks**; these generally fade with time. Others are born with **strawberry marks** (raised red areas with white marks). They often grow a bit before shrinking and they may disappear at about eighteen months. Sometimes children are born with a **skin rash** transmitted from a maternal infection; this may need treatment.
- The **hips** are checked for congenital dislocation of the hip. If present, the baby will be referred to an orthopaedic surgeon for treatment.
- The doctor listens to the baby's **heart** using a stethoscope to ascertain the regularity and the heart sounds. Any abnormalities may suggest congenital heart disease. Blue/purple discoloration of the lips (cyanosis) is associated with some of the serious forms of congenital heart disease. Whilst listening to the heart, the doctor will check that the **femoral pulses** (pulses found in the groin) can be felt, as they may be very difficult to feel in a certain form of congenital heart disease.
- The doctor checks that the **chest** rises and falls symmetrically with inhalation and exhalation. He or she will also listen to the chest with a stethoscope to check there is air entry into both lungs.

12

- The **spine** is checked for evidence of spina bifida (see page 146). This is a condition where one or two of the vertebra (the bones of the spine) have not completely fused together. Children born with evidence of spina bifida will be referred to a surgeon as a matter of some urgency. The spine is also checked for position: it should run down the centre of the back. Any curvature to one side (scoliosis) will need further investigation.
- The baby's **muscle tone** is also assessed. A baby who feels very floppy may have cerebral palsy or Down's syndrome.
- The **anus** is checked for patency (whether it is open or not). This is done when the midwife checks the baby's rectal temperature soon after birth. The midwife is asked to note when meconium (first stool that is passed after birth) is passed; this also confirms that the anus is patent.
- In a boy, the **testes** are felt to determine whether or not they have descended. Undescended testes will usually descend within the first years of life; however, if they do not, surgical intervention will take place, usually before the child starts school. If left undescended, the child may be sterile when he is older, or, in some cases, undescended testes may undergo malignant changes. The opening of the **urethra** is also checked; it should be at the end of the penis (occasionally it opens onto the side of the penis (hypospadia), and surgical intervention may be required).
- In girls, the presence of the **vagina** is checked. Very rarely, the **labia** are fused together, requiring surgery.
- The **temperature** at this time is taken rectally, as it reflects as near to the central core temperature as possible. It is important at this stage to record the temperature, as the child has been delivered from the uterus – where the temperature is 37°C – to a room temperature of approximately 22°C. A new baby has a poorly developed temperature regulating system and a large surface area from which to lose heat and is therefore prone to heat loss and the risk of hypothermia.
- The **umbilical cord** is checked to ensure that three vessels are present (there should be two arteries and one vein).
- The **abdomen** is checked for **hernias**. A hernia is a protrusion of a part of an organ through a weakness in the wall which contains it (for example, hernias are sometimes apparent in the groin). Babies with hernias may be referred to a surgeon. Hernias are often

13

retractable (i.e. they will go back into the abdomen when gentle pressure is placed on them). If the hernia is not retractable, it will require urgent treatment.

- **Limbs** should be symmetrical. Some babies are born with deformities of the lower limbs; the most common of these is talipes, a condition where the foot is not in correct alignment with the leg. These babies need to be referred for orthopaedic advice. The hands are checked for **palmar creases** – two are usually present. The feet are checked for **plantar creases**. In a baby with Down's syndrome, only one palmar and one plantar crease is seen. The number of **digits** on the hands and feet are counted; extra digits are usually removed.

Checklist for Reference

- General appearance.
- Weight.
- Head circumference.
- Fontanelles.
- Mouth.
- Skin.
- Hips.
- Heart.
- Chest.
- Spine.
- Muscle tone.
- Anus.
- Genitalia.
- Temperature.
- Umbilical cord.
- Abdomen.
- Limbs.

HEARING AND LANGUAGE

- It is often very difficult to define whether or not a newborn baby has any hearing loss. However, he or she will 'startle' to sudden loud noises. This reflex is sometimes referred to as the **moro** reflex (see figure 2).
- The baby will have different cries according to his or her needs.

Checklist for Reference

- Hearing: the moro (or startle) reflex.
- Language: the cry.

14

VISION

The child's **eyes** are checked; the **pupils** should be of equal size and should constrict when a light is shone on them. The doctor will reflect a light off the back of the eye; the presence of a red reflex will exclude congenital cataract (an opacity of the lens that prevents the light reaching the back of the eye) and the rare but serious condition, retinoblastoma (a rare tumour of the retina).

Checklist for Reference

- Pupil reaction to light.
- Red reflex.

MOTOR SYSTEM

Reflexes are shown in figure 2 in diagrammatic form so that you can re-familiarise yourself with them.

Rooting reflex	The baby's cheek is touched; he or she will turn the head to locate with the mouth whatever has touched the cheek.	
Grasp reflex	The baby will grasp anything put into his or her hand.	
Stepping reflex	The baby is held up with one foot in contact with a surface. The other foot is brought up as though walking.	
Sucking reflex	The baby will suck on anything put into his or her mouth.	
Moro (or startle) reflex	The baby will fling out the arms when startled. The hands are spread out and then clenched.	

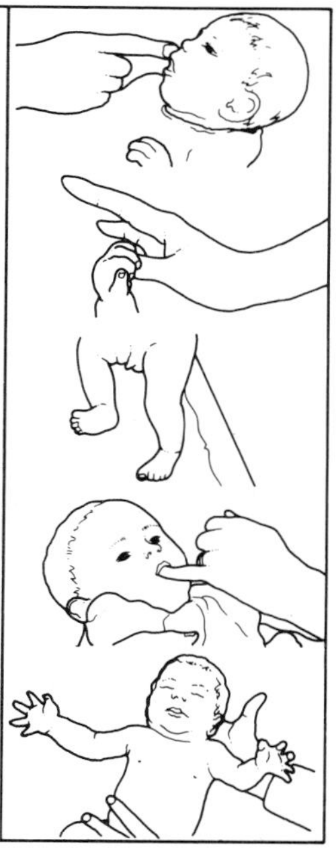

Figure 2   Reflexes – The presence of reflexes are not specially tested but may be observed during the examination.

CARE OF THE SICK CHILD

Checklist for Reference – Reflexes

- The presence of the rooting reflex.
- The presence of the grasping reflex.
- The presence of the stepping reflex.
- The presence of the sucking reflex.
- The presence of the startle (moro) reflex.

The baby's head is floppy and requires support when the baby is lifted. This floppiness of the head is referred to as head lag.

MANIPULATION

The presence of the grasp reflex (see figure 2) demonstrates manipulation.

SOCIAL

When first born, the baby is often alert, will gaze into the mother's face and will also feed vigorously during this time. Later, the newborn baby becomes sleepy.

This concludes the examination at birth. However, if the examining doctor is concerned about any issue, he or she will make arrangements for the child to be followed up by the general practitioner or a specialist.

The midwife will do a blood test (the Guthrie test) when she visits on the sixth day; this is to check that the baby does not have phenylketonuria (see page 136) or hypothyroidism (see page 131).

The community midwife will visit the mother and baby daily until the tenth day. During the postnatal period, the general practitioner may also visit. The health visitor will visit ten to fourteen days after the birth. He or she will give advice on any problems and information about the child surveillance clinics.

The Examination at the Child Surveillance Clinic

The parent will be invited to bring the child into the clinic at the age of six to eight weeks, six to nine months, two years and four and a half years.

THE SIX-TO-EIGHT-WEEK CHECK

Research has shown that the examinations at birth and at six-to-eight weeks show more abnormalities than any other examinations.

This check is usually carried out in the health centre by one of the general practitioners or by the clinical medical officers. Parents will have been reminded to read the page of questions in the Personal Child Health Record Book by the health visitor prior to bringing the baby to the clinic.

The doctor will ask the parent if there have been any problems. These introductory remarks may lead to discussion on anything that may be bothering the parent. The doctor will then perform the examination. While the parent is undressing the baby, the doctor will be observing the baby's reactions and responses, for example smiles, enjoyment, eye contact, plus the ability to undress the baby and any difficulties. These observations give some indication as to how the bonding process is going.

Physical Development

This examination may detect any abnormalities not picked up at birth. Abnormalities may have developed since birth or perhaps they were not obvious at birth. If any abnormalities are detected, they will be discussed with the parents and support will be offered. Any abnormalities are dealt with either by referring the baby to a specialist or by carefully monitoring the situation at regular intervals.

The examination will follow the lines of the examination at birth (refer back to the list on page 14). In addition, the following points are noted and recorded.

- The general **appearance** will give an indication of whether the child is well nourished and appears to have had good care.

17

- The baby will be **weighed** naked, and the weight will be plotted on the growth (or centile) chart. Head circumference will also be measured and plotted.
- The **posterior fontanelle** is usually closed by now. However, the anterior fontanelle does not close until around eighteen months.

At this clinic, the doctor or health visitor may discuss feeding, immunisations and any other concerns the parent may have. Advice on vitamins and fluoride and information on safety may also be given.

Hearing and Language

The parent will be asked if he or she thinks the baby can hear. A baby who can hear will startle to a sudden noise. He or she is often beginning to 'coo' at this stage and will 'freeze' for some sounds.

Vision

The baby will turn his or her head and follow a light, for example the light from a small torch, and will gaze intently into the face of the person who feeds him or her and appear to be studying the face. He or she will often gaze at contrasts. Pupils will constrict when a bright light is shone into them.

Motor System and Manipulation

The baby still has head lag although this is now not so pronounced. When placed prone, he or she will turn the head to one side. The hands are held with the thumbs inwards and the fingers wrapped around them.

Social

The baby is more responsive than when newly born. The feeding pattern usually becomes more regular at this time, and the baby may well be a little more predictable. He or she will stop crying when picked up or when spoken to and look at the person who is talking with great interest. He or she will be smiling by this time.

At the end of the examination, the doctor will record the baby's progress in the Personal Child Health Record Book and invite any questions or problems that the parent may feel need for discussion.

18

THE EXAMINATION AT SIX TO NINE MONTHS

The doctor (or health visitor) will examine the baby and will again observe the mother and baby interaction. Around this age, many children are very clingy; this is to be expected. The examination may therefore take a little longer than previous examinations.

Physical Development

The baby's **head circumference** and **weight** will be measured as before, and the measurements will be plotted on the growth (or centile) charts. A physical examination will be carried out, specifically checking the **hips** and, for boys, the **testes**.

Motor System

The parent will be asked if the child can sit and roll, both of which are usually within the capabilities of the eight-month-old child. Muscle tone will be observed, particularly when the child is sitting on the mother's lap. He or she will often want to stand and hold on to the parent and push with the feet.

Manipulation

During the assessment, the baby will be offered a toy, which is usually taken in one hand and then passed to the other. He or she will be observed for equal use of the hands and for accuracy with passing and grasping. At this stage, some babies can use a pincer grasp, which can be demonstrated by inviting the baby to pick up 'hundreds and thousands' (these can safely be put into the mouth, which is the usual response).

Vision

The parent will be asked specifically about the child's eyesight. Whilst the child is playing, visual behaviour will be observed and he or she will be checked for any signs of a squint which, if present, will require referral to an ophthalmologist (eye specialist).

Hearing

The parent will be asked if he or she thinks the baby can hear. It is important that any hearing loss should be picked up early, because it can lead to language and learning difficulties. Any family history of hearing

19

loss will be noted. A hearing defect may not be readily picked up by the parents, and therefore all children are screened for hearing loss using a distraction test (see below).

Distraction Test

The distraction test is carried out between seven and eight months. It is essential that the test is carried out in a quiet room and that there are two people present to carry out the test.

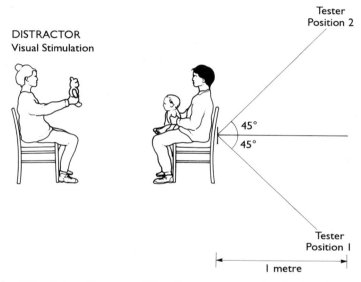

Figure 3   The distraction test   The distractor uses visual stimulation to gain the child's attention. Only when the child is looking at the stimulator will the tester make a sound. The same sound is made from each side, as shown. A range of sounds is tested.

The aim of the test is to see if the child hears sounds of varying sound and pitch. As shown in figure 3, the test is carried out from both sides so that it can be ascertained if the child has hearing in both ears. The child is tested at one metre from each ear. He or she sits on the parent's lap, and the helper presents a distraction so that the child is concentrating on something other than the person producing the sound. Once the child is concentrating, the distractor reduces the distraction and the person testing the hearing will now produce a sound one metre from one ear and then one metre from the other ear.

20

If the child fails the distraction test, the health visitor will usually arrange to repeat the test approximately one month later. It is worth noting that a baby may fail if he or she has a cold or ear infection. If the child fails again, he or she is referred to an audiologist (a person trained to assess hearing).

Language

The parent will be asked about any sounds the baby makes; he or she is usually 'cooling' at this stage and often chattering tunefully using consonant sounds. He or she may shout to attract attention and will listen and then shout again. The child is often able to recognise voices, particularly his or her parents, and will usually listen when spoken to and may even try to carry on the 'conversation'.

Children who are deaf *do* vocalise, but these vocalisations remain at a basic level. A child who has not developed these tuneful repetitive sounds by the age of eight or nine months is investigated for possible deafness. Children who have an undetected hearing loss may show behavioural problems, which usually disappear quickly once the hearing loss has been corrected.

THE TWO-YEAR CHECK

This check follows the pattern of the previous tests. The parent will be asked some general questions about his or her own health and that of the baby. Any worries will be discussed.

Physical Development

This follows the lines of the previous examinations. If the doctor is concerned about any findings, the child will be referred to the appropriate specialist. It is worth noting that, if the testes have not yet descended, the boy will be referred to a paediatric surgeon for an opinion, and undescended testes usually are operated on before the child starts school.

Vision

The parent is specifically asked if he or she has observed anything to suggest the child cannot see. The child is referred to an ophthalmologist (eye specialist) if necessary.

Language

The parent is asked about the child's speech. The child generally has an average vocabulary of 200 understandable words at this stage. He or she is able to join two words together and is continually questioning.

Hearing

The parent will be asked if he or she has any worries about the child's hearing. If there are any problems, the child will probably be referred for a hearing test and possibly for a specialist opinion. Treatment will be given as necessary.

Social

Potty training is usually underway at this stage. Some children may be clean and dry in the day (and possibly at night), while others are still in nappies. The doctor or health visitor is usually willing to discuss training and give help and guidance as necessary. The child may throw temper tantrums when frustrated – the 'terrible twos'. This can sometimes be distressing for the parent, and problems will be discussed as necessary. The child will probably play near other children but not with them yet. He or she is becoming increasingly independent but is obviously still very dependent on an adult.

Motor System

At this stage, the child is usually walking with a normal gait (manner of walking), can often manage stairs holding on to the rail and two feet to a step, runs and can use push-and-pull toys.

Manipulation

The child can build a tower of six or seven bricks, can hold a pencil using the thumb and two fingers and can turn the pages of a book one page at a time.

THE PRE-SCHOOL CHECK (USUALLY AT FOUR-AND-A-HALF)

The aim of this check, which is carried out by a doctor, is to see if there are any problems not yet detected that might interfere with the child's education. The parent is asked if he or she has any worries, and these are discussed as necessary. He or she is specifically asked if the child has any problems that might affect schooling.

Physical Development

The child's **height** and **weight** are measured and plotted on the growth (centile) chart. The heart is listened to for any abnormal sounds (the child would be referred to a cardiologist if any abnormalities were detected). In a boy, the **testes** will be checked again (if they have not descended, the child will be referred to a surgeon).

Motor System

The child can usually walk up and downstairs using one foot to a stair, walk on tiptoe, hop, stand on one foot and then the other.

Manipulation

The child has good control of pencils and paintbrushes and can draw and colour pictures.

Language

The child is usually fairly fluent and can recite short rhymes. He or she may be asked to name objects drawn on a language board.

Hearing and Vision

If the parent has any worries about the child's ability to hear or see, the child will be referred to the appropriate specialist.

Social

The child is more independent and can usually dress and undress, use a knife and fork, and wash his or her hands and face. He or she is usually clean and dry throughout the day and night, although the child may still have accidents at night. He or she usually has some friends and will play with them.

At all of these clinic appointments, opportunities are taken to discuss health education topics. These include safety and the prevention of accidents, nutrition, dental care, care of the child in the sun and smoking and the adverse effects on the child.

Immunisations

At each clinic, the doctor will check that the child has had the relevant immunisations and will discuss any apprehensions that the parents may have, presenting the factual information to the parents so that they can make up their own minds. (This is an important skill for carers to follow, as they may often be asked advice on issues. Presenting information in a factual way allows parents to make up their own minds and means that they have played an active part in the decision making and are therefore responsible for making an informed decision.) Parents are asked to sign a consent form prior to immunisations being given.

Note: BCG (Bacillus Calmette-Guerin) is recommended for all infants born to parents who are immigrants from countries where tuberculosis is of high prevalence (for example, the Indian subcontinent). It is given within the first few days of life after the consent form has been signed by a parent.

Immunisations are only given if the child is well. (They will be postponed if he or she is unwell.) The doctor will ask if he or she has had any reaction to a previous immunisation and will check that the child is not taking medication (or has an illness) which interferes with the ability to fight infection.

CARE OF THE CHILD AFTER IMMUNISATION

The child should be kept cool; his or her temperature may rise slightly in the few days after the immunisation. Ensure that he or she has plenty of fluids, and if he or she might becomes hot and irritable, a bath in slightly cooler water than usual is recommended. The child should be patted dry (not rubbed) afterwards. If he or she is still hot and irritable, paediatric paracetamol in the dose prescribed should be given. If the carer is worried, he or she should ring the doctor.

IMMUNISATION SCHEDULE

two months:	diphtheria pertussis tetanus	} given as a single injection
	HIB	given in another site
	polio	given orally
three months:	diphtheria pertussis tetanus	} given as a single injection
	HIB	given in another site
	polio	given orally
four months:	diphtheria pertussis tetanus	} given as a single injection
	HIB	given in another site
	polio	given orally
twelve–eighteen months:	measles mumps rubella	} (MMR) given as a single injection
four–five years:	diphtheria tetanus	} given as a single injection
	polio	given orally
ten–fourteen years:	rubella BCG	given to girls only (Bacillus Calmette-Guerin vaccine) given as an injection to give protection against tuberculosis. (This is not given in all regions)
fifteen–eighteen years:	tetanus diphtheria	} booster, given as single injection
	polio	booster, given orally

3

RECOGNISING THE ILL CHILD

—

Adults tend to tell anyone and everyone if they are feeling unwell. This is really a request for sympathy and tolerance. Young children do not have the communication skills and knowledge from past experiences to warn their carers that they feel unwell. Carers should therefore be aware of the possible signs and symptoms of illness. Carers are often practised in the art of observation. This skill eventually becomes second nature and serves as a good grounding for child care, enabling the carer to be sensitive to the child's needs.

Clues that a Child is Unwell

BEHAVIOURAL CHANGES

Behavioural changes may be apparent when a child is unwell. He or she may be quieter than usual, more clingy, appear to be attention-seeking or perhaps whining and irritable. The sleep pattern may alter, with some sleeping more than usual and others sleeping less. The child may be less energetic or appear to regress (behave as if he or she were younger).

Carers should always remind themselves that these features are related to the child's inability to tell the carer the problem, and that they often precede an illness.

The child may show less interest in his or her toys or choose toys that he or she had previously outgrown. Ill children often like to watch television or videos, as these require less effort.

COMMUNICATION

The carer will usually be able to pick up the fact that the child is in pain from verbal and/or non-verbal clues. Sometimes assessing the severity of the pain may be difficult.

- Crying: a baby may cry more than usual. The carer will often be able to detect different cries, for example those of hunger or pain. A characteristically high-pitched cry may be heard in a baby with meningitis. A baby who is whimpering may be exhausted. An older child may also cry, but be unable to explain the reason.
- Verbal clues: some children can give an indication of the problem, but this will depend on the child's age and stage of development: for example, a four-year-old may say that he or she has a headache, but point to the abdomen.
- Non-verbal clues: these can be good indicators that a child is unwell. The carer should look at the face, the position the child has adopted, movement (which may be limited), and sometimes an injured arm or leg may be protectively held.

PHYSICAL SIGNS

Colour

If the child has a raised temperature, the face may be flushed. An ill child (without a raised temperature) often has a pale appearance. If the child has difficulty breathing, he or she may appear blue at the extremities, such as the fingernails, or may even have a blue appearance centrally, for example, inside the lips (which can be seen to be pink in all people, regardless of ethnic origin). A yellow tinge may be seen in jaundiced children, particularly on the sclera (white of the eye) or under the tongue.

Expression

The expression may indicate discomfort or pain.

Mouth

The lips may be dry or cracked, the tongue may be coated, the breath may smell, the mucous membrane inside the mouth may have white patches on it, the gums may show evidence of infection, i.e. swelling or even pus. The child may be breathing through the mouth, which is obviously significant if the child normally breathes through the nose.

Nose

There may be nasal discharge, the quantity and colour of which may be of importance, for example thick and green, clear or bloody.

Eyes

There may be a discharge of pus if there is an infection, and the eyes may look red. The child may also be rubbing them because they itch or if he or she has been crying. Photophobia (dislike of light) may be suggested by turning away from bright windows or by verbally protesting if the light is turned on.

Ears

There may be a permanent or intermittent hearing loss. Pain may be suggested by the child touching or rubbing the ear(s). A pustular, sometimes smelly, discharge may be seen with an acute infection. After a head injury, there may be a straw-coloured discharge from either the ear or nose, indicating a loss of cerebro-spinal fluid.

Skin

The colour changes have been outlined above. Skin rashes may be seen in some infectious and allergic conditions. The distribution and colour will vary according to the cause. Bruising is often seen in young children and is partly due to the nature of their unsteadiness and is commonly seen on the shins. However, excessive bruising, particularly in unusual areas such as the trunk, bottom and back, may suggest illness, such as leukaemia, or child abuse. Skin has an elasticity which it tends to lose when dehydrated through illness.

Respiratory Tract

The child's cough may be described as wheezy (i.e. a high-pitched whistling noise heard when the child breathes out (exhalation)), productive (i.e. the child coughs up some sputum or phlegm which is usually swallowed), dry (non-productive), barking (sounds like a dog's bark), or a characteristic whoop may be heard when the child breathes in (inhalation).

The cough may be worse at night. The child may be distressed by the constant coughing or may appear to accept the situation. The carer should be aware of the child's normal respiratory rate, which is often increased when the child has a cough. A grunting sound may be heard when the child breathes. The carer may notice that the muscles between the ribs appear to be sucked in. This is typically seen in a severe asthmatic attack.

Renal System

The child may pass urine more frequently than usual. If dehydrated the child will pass little urine. It may be painful to pass urine; the urine may smell or appear cloudy if infected. The previously potty-trained child may be incontinent more often than would usually be accepted as the 'odd accident'.

Gastro-Intestinal System

Ill children generally have a decreased appetite and are usually fussier with their food. Changes in bowel habits may be apparent, with the child perhaps developing constipation or diarrhoea. Vomiting may be associated with a number of conditions. The amount and consistency are important. Any blood in vomit or in stools should be reported to the doctor.

Nervous System

The conscious level may alter in some circumstances, for example after a head injury. The carer should be aware of the importance of seeking medical help should this occur. The following terms refer to levels of consciousness: fully conscious – alert and responsive; unconscious – unaware of surroundings and not rousable. Between these levels the child may be unusually drowsy and may, perhaps, slur their speech.

Temperature

A child may develop a raised temperature as a result of an infection. The child may be flushed in the face and feel hot, thirsty and irritable. If the temperature becomes very high, he or she may hallucinate and become very agitated. There is a possibility that he or she will go on to have a febrile convulsion.

A hypothermic child, on the other hand, may be cold to the touch, have a flushed face despite the cold temperature, appear to be immobile and have shallow breathing.

The carer should note that the ill child's signs and symptoms tend to build up gradually over several hours or days, however, in some circumstances, they appear acutely.

When to Seek Medical Advice

Medical advice should be sought if the child:

- has a raised temperature and other signs of illness;
- feels hot and appears to have neck stiffness and/or dislike of light;
- feels cold and is listless;
- feels cold and sweaty;
- has a fit (convulsion) – this may be accompanied by a raised temperature;
- has any difficulty breathing, for example, choking, wheezing;
- has a barking cough;
- cannot breathe freely;
- has breathing that sounds like grunting;
- is too breathless to talk;
- appears to be sucking in his or her ribs (rib recession) and has a problem with breathing;
- complains of pain on breathing;
- coughs up blood;
- is drowsy or difficult to rouse and/or does not recognise people;
- is unusually quiet or listless;
- is in pain;
- cries for an unusually long time (enough to arouse suspicion that he or she be in pain);
- keeps refusing food or drink;
- has frequent loose stools, especially if they contain blood;
- vomits and/or has diarrhoea for more than six hours (particularly important if the child is under two years old);
- vomits blood;
- vomits and appears to be in pain;
- has recently had a head injury and feels sick or vomits, or experiences a change of conscious level or if the pupils are no longer equal in size;
- is unable to use any part of his or her body;
- has a suspected fracture;
- will not feed or suck (young baby).

It is difficult to consider every situation. If a carer is worried about the health of any child in his or her care, medical advice should be sought from the GP or the health visitor, who will often be happy to give telephone advice. It may be suggested that the child is brought to the surgery where he or she will usually be seen quickly, and any examination or tests can be carried out with the facilities available.

EMERGENCIES

Call an ambulance immediately. If possible, call a doctor as well, as he or she will often get there before the ambulance and may know the child's history and can therefore initiate treatment. The child should not be given anything to eat or drink until seen by the doctor.

Emergencies are when the child:

- stops breathing;
- is having difficulty breathing and is going blue (he or she may appear 'waxy');
- is unconscious;
- is bleeding and it cannot be controlled;
- has eaten or drunk any toxic substance, such as bleach;
- has sustained a serious burn;
- has a chemical in his or her eyes;
- is in any situation where life is at risk.

Role of the Carer

When any child is unwell, the carer should carry out the following procedure:

1 Inform the next-of-kin. It is imperative that you have a contact number. If the child needs to be seen as an emergency, medical advice needs to be sought first. Inform the next-of-kin once the initial danger has passed.

2 On the instructions of the next-of-kin, arrange for a doctor to see the child. This will involve telephoning the surgery to request an appointment.

While the child is being examined, the carer should:

3 Stay with the child at all times. This is reassuring to the child and allows the carer to assist if necessary.

4 Prepare the child as much as possible. Remember the child is feeling unwell and may be a little irritable and frightened. When talking to the child, use language that he or she understands and try not to be in a rush.

5 Assist the doctor as necessary.

6 Undress the child, as appropriate, after asking his or her permission.

7 Give the history of the illness to the doctor clearly and concisely. Be accurate in the description, include your observations and any other information thought necessary. Don't be afraid to offer an opinion, for example, 'I think he may have an ear infection', or to clarify points.

8 Include past medical history, particularly if the doctor is not the usual doctor.

9 When the examination is over, the doctor will give some explanation and probably some instructions. Clarify the information and write it down if necessary (you will need to relay the information to the parents). The following information will be needed: the diagnosis, the treatment, additional instructions, how the child reacted and the date and time of any follow-up.

10 Take the child home, unless an admission to hospital is necessary. Reassure the child. Allow him or her to rest. Follow the instructions given.

EXAMINATION OF THE CHILD

The examination will depend to some extent on the history given and may involve some of the following:

• The child's temperature may be taken.
• Palpation for swollen glands. Lymph glands may swell when there is an infection; their detection will help in the diagnosis (see figure 4).
• An examination of the ear may take place. The child will be shown the auroscope and positioned as shown in figure 5. This will enable the doctor to examine him or her as quickly as possible and with the minimum distress.
• An examination of the eye will involve a general observation of the inflammation and infection (as in conjunctivitis), or it may be a

32

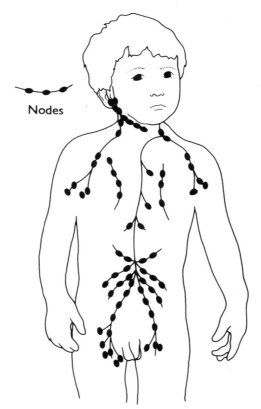

Nodes

Figure 4   The lymphatic system

more detailed examination of the back of the eye using an
ophthalmoscope or the instillation of some drops to assist the
examination.

• For an examination of the throat, position the child as shown in
  figure 6. Young children find the examination of the throat slightly
  unpleasant, but a securely held child, held as shown in the diagram,
  enables the doctor to get a good view of the throat and to complete
  the procedure as quickly as possible.

• During the examination the doctor will observe the skin for rashes,
  colour and general appearance. He or she may ask questions about
  any observations.

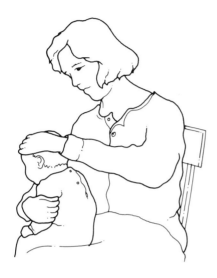

Figure 5   Examination of the ear   The doctor will use an auroscope to look into the ear. Position the child to one side. Make him or her comfortable. Hold both arms by the side and gently hold the head steady. After examination of one ear, turn the child the other way.

Figure 6   Examination of the throat   Position the child facing the doctor. Gently restrain the arms at the side and support the head. The doctor will ask the child to open the mouth and will then depress the tongue to gain a good view of the throat with the aid of a torch. Note that this procedure is often disliked.

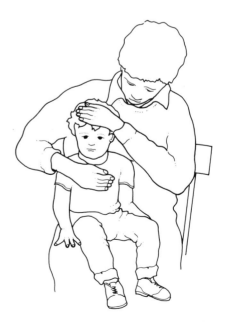

34

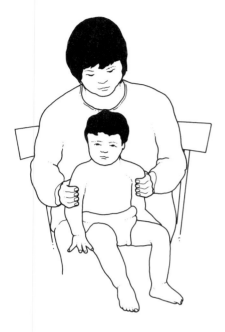

Figure 7   Examination of the chest   Position the child on the carer's lap, facing the doctor. Hold the arms at the side.

Figure 8   Examination of the chest   Position the child to one side so that the doctor may listen to the back of the chest.

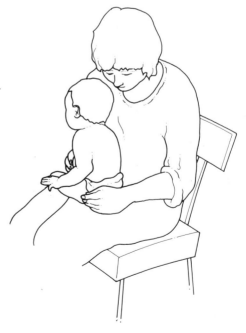

- It will be necessary to remove the child's outer clothing and lift their vest to examine the chest. A small child is usually examined sitting on the carer's lap. An older child will sit on a chair. The doctor will often let a small child play with the stethoscope before putting it on the chest so that he or she is familiar with it. During this time, the doctor will be noting the respiratory rate and observing the chest to check, for example, for rib recession. He or she will then listen to the front and the back of the chest for air entry into the lungs and then count the heart rate (see figures 7 and 8).
- For the examination of the abdomen, a young baby may be more easily examined sitting on the carer's lap. An older child should lie on the bed or couch as shown in figure 9.
- If meningitis is a possibility, the doctor may examine the child for neck stiffness. The child should be positioned on his or her back (see figure 10).
- If a fracture or sprain is suspected, the doctor may look at the affected limb and then compare it with the other limb. Any swelling is then more obvious.

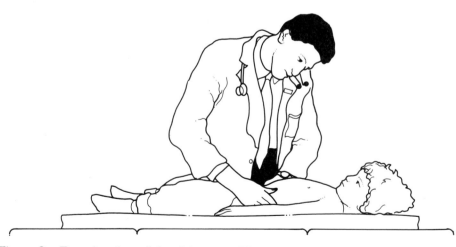

Figure 9   Examination of the abdomen   The child is asked to lie on the couch in the prone position. The carer should stay with the child to ensure safety and to reassure him or her.

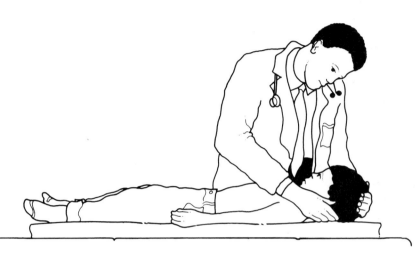

Figure 10   Examination for neck stiffness   The child will lie prone without a pillow. The doctor will tell the child to relax while holding the head. The head will then be lifted up and forwards. A child with neck stiffness will resist this. The carer should stay near the child to ensure safety and to reassure him or her.

STUDENT ACTIVITY

Role of the Carer

I   Under the heading *The role of the carer*, you were instructed to inform the next-of-kin. Work in pairs and role-play the following situation:

A three-year-old child in the day nursery has developed a raised temperature during the morning and has become increasingly unwell. The nearest parent works in the next town and the supervisor has decided that the parent should be informed and suggested that the child should be taken home.

For the purpose of this role-play, one of you takes the part of the parent and the other the supervisor. You will need to plan the conversation first. What will you say to the parent? How will you introduce the information?

Consider the impact on the parent of being telephoned and told the child is unwell. It may not be convenient for the parent to leave work at that moment; how will you persuade them that it is in the child's best interests? How will you record the conversation?

4

Principles of Caring for Ill Children

___

Ill children need their parents or regular carer. During illness, they need the security and extra attention of the people they trust the most. It is these people that can provide the understanding and patience necessary.

Children do not like being separated from their familiar carers when they are unwell, and generally childminders or day nurseries do not encourage parents to leave ill children.

The Needs of the Ill Child

Children react to illness in different ways, depending on many factors, such as age and developmental stage, family expectations, understanding and cultural background. Caring for children, whether well or sick, requires the carer to meet their needs. Although considered here under separate headings, they are interlinked.

COMFORT

Changes in the child's life, including illness, may lead to feelings of insecurity. It is the responsibility of the parents and carers to help overcome these feelings by showing understanding and sympathy. Reassurance and comfort help to provide the security in times of stress. This can be achieved by:

- caring for the child in his or her own surroundings, and ideally by their parent(s) or regular carer;
- nursing the child in a room near the family;
- using language the child will understand to explain the situation;
- accepting that regression is common in the circumstances;

- always telling the truth – this will ensure trust;
- giving plenty of time and attention;
- telling the child that he or she will soon be well again (unless this is obviously not the case);
- ensuring that, if the child is admitted to hospital, a parent stays too, if possible.

DRINKS

A good fluid intake will help to reduce a raised temperature and will prevent dehydration, so children should be encouraged to drink plenty of fluids when they are unwell. This can be achieved by tempting them with fluids that are usually only offered on special occasions, such as Coca-Cola or ice lollies. Sometimes children will gain comfort by using the bottle or a feeder cup that they have recently grown out of.

FOOD

A small child's appetite usually decreases when ill. Small amounts of attractively arranged food should be offered.

Some conditions, such as diabetes and cystic fibrosis, require a special diet, and the dietician will usually meet the parents/carers to explain about the diet; specific instructions should be followed.

REST AND SLEEP

A sick child requires more rest and sleep than usual. The child will often be the best guide to the amount needed. When asleep, he or she will need to be checked regularly to monitor his or her condition. A paediatric community nurse may be available for advice on home nursing and prevention of the complications of bedrest for more long-term cases.

PLAY AND ACTIVITY

Play is an essential part of normal development for any child. Regression will often mean that he or she prefers to play in the way that he or she did at a younger age. The child should be allowed to gain as much enjoyment as possible to distract them from the illness. Play and its possible implications need to be thought through; for instance, painting when in bed does require the undivided attention of a responsible adult.

If a child has periods of feeling better and wants to go outside to play, this is acceptable as long as the weather is suitable. He or she will need to be dressed appropriately and supervised at all times. **N.B. Children with infectious diseases should not play with other children who have not had the disease.**

HYGIENE

An ill child will feel more comfortable if he or she is washed regularly. A daily bath is not essential, although it may be enjoyed by some children. The child's hands, face and bottom should be washed at least twice a day. Teeth should be cleaned at the same time. Clothes and bedclothes will need to be changed and washed more frequently than usual. The carer must maintain a high standard of personal hygiene at all times.

ELIMINATION

Bowel habits often change during an illness, and medical advice may be necessary. Constipation may be avoided by ensuring the child has a good fluid intake and eats some fruit and vegetables. The urinary output may decrease, as the body loses fluid if the temperature is raised. If the urinary output is absent or very low, then medical advice should be sought. In babies, this is clearly indicated by dry nappies.

If the child has diarrhoea or is incontinent, he or she will need reassurance, and the area should be carefully washed and dried and a barrier cream applied. Clean clothes should be put on.

FRESH AIR

Good ventilation is essential, and the window may be opened to circulate fresh air.

SAFETY

Safety is of paramount importance. The carer will need:

- to observe for unwanted effects of treatment and report this to the doctor;
- to be aware of any specific complications of the illness or medication;

- to know how to use equipment safely;
- may need to stay with the child at night so that he or she can be closely watched.

MEDICAL CARE

See page 30 for when to seek medical advice and page 51 for advice on medication.

Medication must be given as directed. A knowledge of common unwanted effects should be known and if there is any evidence of unwanted effects they must be reported to the doctor.

If the child's condition deteriorates or if the carer is worried about the child, he or she should consult a doctor. If admission to hospital seems likely, the carer should prepare the child (see page 154).

SOCIAL CONTACT

When the child is unwell, he or she will probably only want his or her carers near. As he or she improves, visits from others are usually enjoyed. These visits may not be possible if the child is infectious. If the child is unwell for a long time and is at school or pre-school, the teacher may arrange for the other children to write, and this can act as a morale booster.

CULTURAL DIFFERENCES

The carer will need to familiarise him or herself with any cultural differences which may affect the care given to the child. The parents will usually give guidelines on issues such as these, and the carer must ensure that he or she is aware of them.

WARMTH

Overheating or underheating can both have serious consequences. The recommended room temperature for a newborn baby is between 18°C and 21°C. As the child grows and the temperature regulating system becomes established, room temperatures can be decreased slightly. Children should be clothed adequately so they feel comfortable in the surroundings.

Temperature Control

Normal body temperature is 37°C (98.4°F). However, there is a normal range of 36°C–37°C. A body temperature over 37.5°C is called a fever or **pyrexia** ('a temperature'). A body temperature of 35°C or less is called **hypothermia**. Remember that temperatures quoted are temperatures that have been taken orally; a temperature taken under the axilla (armpit) is slightly lower than an oral (mouth) temperature (by approximately 0.5°C).

Body temperature does vary slightly throughout the day, and it is usually found to be slightly higher in the evening. If you suspect that a child in your care has a raised temperature, you should measure it. If a doctor's advice is to be sought, he or she may ask for the temperature reading, and it is helpful to be specific.

THERMOMETERS

There are several types of thermometer available; the most commonly used is the mercury thermometer. Others include the digital thermometer and the fever strip. The digital thermometer is slightly more expensive, but has the advantages of being easily read and less hazardous because it is not made of glass. The fever strip is easy to use, but due to its lack of sensitivity it is not recommended.

TAKING A CHILD'S TEMPERATURE

In order to take the child's temperature, the following sequence should be followed:

- collect the equipment;
- find books or toys that can be used as distractions;
- use language that the child will understand and tell him or her what you are going to do, as you will require his or her co-operation;
- sit the child on your knee.

Using a Digital Thermometer under the Arm

- Take the thermometer out of its case and place it under the arm as shown in figure 11.
- The thermometer should be read when the temperature stops rising.

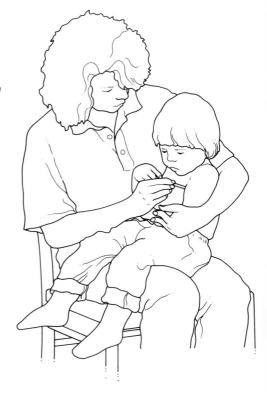

Figure 11   Taking the axillary temperature   The parent or carer sits with the child on the lap. A mercury thermometer is shaken until the mercury is below the reading of 35°C. A digital thermometer needs no preparation. The thermometer is placed under the child's arm and held there while the reading is taken. It may help to distract the child's attention during this process.

Using a Mercury Thermometer

- Shake the mercury in the thermometer down to the bottom of the thermometer.
- Place the thermometer under the child's arm.
- Hold the child as shown in figure 11, thus protecting the thermometer from breaking.
- Read to the child or play in this limited position until the thermometer has finally measured the temperature (this may take up to five minutes).

Remember, never leave a child alone with a mercury thermometer – it is made of glass, which could break, and it contains mercury which, if exposed, could be a health hazard.

HYPOTHERMIA

Hypothermia describes the state when the child's body temperature drops below 35°C.

Babies are prone to hypothermia for several reasons:

- they have a relatively large surface area from which to lose heat;
- they are unable to shiver, so they cannot easily regain their body temperature once it has dropped;
- they are relatively inactive and therefore depend on their carer to dress them adequately for their environment;
- their temperature regulating system is poorly developed.

Hypothermia can be fatal. If the carer suspects that a child may be hypothermic, a low-reading thermometer will need to be used. If one is not available and hypothermia is suspected, there is no time for delay – medical help should be requested immediately.

How to Recognise the Hypothermic Child

- The child is cold to the touch. This is because the blood vessels to the skin have constricted (vasoconstriction) in an attempt to conserve heat. If the carer suspects that the child has hypothermia, a good indicator is to feel the child's abdomen or under the arms, both of which usually feel warm.
- The child appears pale (sometimes the face does appear to be flushed). This occurs because the body is trying to maintain an even temperature to the core of the body so that the vital functions are maintained.
- If the child is conscious, he or she may be confused and his or her speech slurred. This occurs because tissue metabolism has altered due to the cold.
- He or she may be drowsy.
- He or she may be shivering. This is unlikely to be seen in a baby, as stated earlier. However, shivering does occur in the older child in an attempt to produce heat.

45

Treatment

It is *vitally important* that the child is warmed slowly. Rapid rewarming will result in the blood vessels to the skin dilating, and the child will then lose more heat. If he or she is wet, remove the wet clothing and wrap him or her in a dry blanket. If the clothes are dry, wrap the child in a blanket and, if possible, a space blanket (a foil-like sheet). These work by preventing further heat loss. If the child is held closely to the carer, he or she will warm up slowly. Call a doctor or an ambulance.

THE CARE OF THE CHILD WITH A FEVER (RAISED TEMPERATURE OR PYREXIA)

The child with a raised temperature will often appear to be irritable and miserable. He or she will often become more clingy or will perhaps appear to be cross. He or she will usually be flushed and hot and perhaps more thirsty than usual.

It is important to reduce a pyrexia in a child, because reduction of the high temperature itself will enable the child to feel a lot better and reduce the risk of a febrile convulsion (see page 48).

Methods of Reducing the Temperature

Cool the Child

Children lose heat through their skin, so keeping them wrapped up means that the heat cannot be lost. If the child is in bed, remove some of the bedclothes. If he or she is dressed, remove some of his or her clothes (remember to ask the child's permission). An infant may be left in a vest and nappy and a child in his or her underclothes. Cotton is the ideal choice, as it is cool to wear. Careful observation of the child will allow the carer to be aware if the child is becoming too cool and some of the clothes need to be replaced.

Give the Child Plenty of Fluids

The child will be hot and feel thirsty. The carer should offer plenty of cold fluids, which will help to reduce the temperature. A toddler or child should be offered cold drinks regularly (at least hourly) and encouraged to take them. Ice lollies are often very popular with pyrexial children, and they are an excellent way of providing the fluids and cooling the child.

A breast-fed baby can be put to the breast more often. He or she will usually suck readily if thirsty.

A bottle-fed baby may be offered boiled, cooled water (slightly flavoured if necessary) at frequent intervals. Milk should be offered according to the usual routine.

Medicines

Paracetamol preparations are medicines that are very efficient at reducing the temperature in a child. They can be bought at the chemist and should always be stored in a locked medicine cupboard. Remember that medicines must not be given unless the permission of the next-of-kin is obtained; ideally this permission should be in writing. (See chapter 5 for information on the giving of medicines.)

Aspirin – or any medicine containing aspirin – should not be given to children under the age of twelve years.

Elixirs or syrups are recommended for young children (or older children who have difficulty swallowing tablets). Medicines should always be given following the instructions.

Paracetamol preparations should not be given to babies under the age of three months unless advised by a doctor or health visitor.

Tepid sponging

This is a method used to reduce a child's temperature if it is very high, i.e. over 38.5°C, particularly if the child is irritable or if there is a history of febrile convulsion. Tepid sponging must be carried out in a draught-free room, using the following procedure.

- Tell the child what you are going to do. Use language that he or she will understand and speak to him or her kindly. Tell the child that the sponging will make him or her feel more comfortable.
- The child can remain in his or her underclothes. Pour water into a bowl. The temperature of the water should be a few degrees lower than the temperature of the child. Use two or three sponges. Place a damp sponge under each armpit and with the other damp sponge gently wipe the child's skin. Leave a layer of moisture on the skin.
- Sometimes an older child may prefer to have a cool bath. Run a bath of warm water a few degrees lower than the temperature of the child. Put him or her in the water and stay with him or her. This has the effect of cooling the child and making him or her feel more

47

comfortable. Take him or her out after a few minutes and gently pat the skin dry.

It is important to watch the child carefully, because if he or she cools too quickly, he or she may start to shiver, which will increase the temperature again.

Remember, you should offer the child a choice of these methods once he or she is old enough to make a choice.

FEBRILE CONVULSIONS

A febrile convulsion is a fit which occurs as a result of a rise in temperature. If a child has had one convulsion, there is an increased risk of having another, and it is therefore important that care is taken to try to reduce the temperature if the child becomes pyrexial again. A child having a febrile convulsion will become rigid, and then the body will start to jerk and twitch. This will only last a short time (one or two minutes). Some children are incontinent of urine or faeces during a convulsion. When the convulsion appears to be over, the child may wake and then sleep, or go straight to sleep. You should do the following:

- place the child in the recovery position (see figure 12);

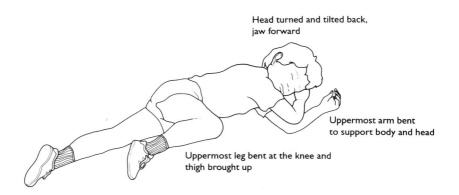

Head turned and tilted back, jaw forward

Uppermost arm bent to support body and head

Uppermost leg bent at the knee and thigh brought up

Figure 12   The recovery position

- stay with the child while he or she is having the convulsion; do not try to control the jerky movements and do not put anything in the mouth; however, if there is already something in the mouth, it must be removed, as there is a risk of choking;
- loosen all tight clothing;
- call the doctor once the convulsion is over;
- start to cool the child by removing some of the layers of clothes.

STUDENT ACTIVITIES

1   You are currently working in a day nursery and you know that two of the children are prone to febrile convulsions when their temperature rises. Prepare a poster for the day nursery giving step-by-step guidelines for the management of children having a febrile convulsion.

2   You are caring for a five-year-old child who has been kept away from school today because he has a heavy cold. Using the information from this chapter, give a written account of how you will meet this child's needs.

3   You are caring for a four-year-old child who has been vomiting for four hours. Using the information from this chapter, give a written account of how you might meet this child's needs.

5

MEDICATION

—

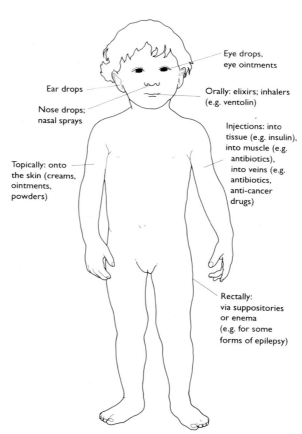

Eye drops,
eye ointments

Ear drops

Orally: elixirs; inhalers
(e.g. ventolin)

Nose drops;
nasal sprays

Injections: into
tissue (e.g. insulin),
into muscle (e.g.
antibiotics),
into veins (e.g.
antibiotics,
anti-cancer
drugs)

Topically: onto
the skin (creams,
ointments,
powders)

Rectally:
via suppositories
or enema
(e.g. for some
forms of epilepsy)

Figure 13   Administration of medication

Medicines fall into two categories: those that can only be prescribed by a doctor and those that can be bought over the counter.

The carer is advised to obtain written and signed permission from a parent before giving the medicine, to avoid possible misunderstandings later. This written permission should include the following details:

- the name of the medicine;
- when it was last given;
- when it is to be given next;
- by which route it should be given, for example by mouth or via an inhaler;
- in the case of medicines that are given 'as necessary', the parent should identify the signs or symptoms the child might show to indicate that the medicine is required: for example, with a paracetamol elixir (to lower the temperature), the parent may suggest that it is only given if the temperature rises above 37.5°C.

The carer should record the time and dose of medicine given. This information can then be given to the parent on their return. Some day-care establishments have specific rules about the administration of medicines, and the carer should familiarise him or herself with the policies.

The medicine should be clearly labelled with the name of the medication, the child's name and the dosage, together with the maximum number of times a day that it can be given. It should be kept out of the reach of children, preferably in a locked medicine cupboard, unless it must be kept in a fridge (which should also, ideally, be lockable).

Medicine are usually given between one and four times a day, some medicines must be taken with or after food. It is important to space the dosages out as far as possible. It is not usually a good idea to wake a child to give the medicine (unless instructed to do so by a doctor), as sleep is beneficial to the ill child.

If the carer is working with several children, it is important that he or she correctly identifies the child and gives him or her the correct medicine; it may be necessary to take along another carer to act as a witness, if this is the policy of the establishment. This should not seem intimidating to the child, since many activities are done with more than one carer.

Always prepare the child. This can be done by:

- telling him or her what you are going to do before the event;
- always use language that he or she will understand;
- be quietly persuasive, but try to see the event from his or her point of view and empathise with him or her: 'I know it's not convenient now, but you will get better more quickly if we do what the doctor said'.

Medication given by Mouth (Orally)

Medicines are usually dispensed in liquid form (elixirs) for children under the age of twelve. The liquid is flavoured to make it as pleasant as possible. The medicines should be shaken before the dose is measured. The dosage of a medicine prescribed by a doctor will be clearly stated. The dosage of a non-prescribed medicine will vary with the age of the child. It is vitally important that these doses are given as directed, both in terms of amount and frequency. Medicines should be poured with the label uppermost so that it is not obliterated if a drop of the medicine runs down the side of the bottle.

When the dose is 5 ml (or a multiple of 5 ml), a 5 ml spoon is provided with the medicine. When the dose is less than 5 ml, a liquid measure is given.

ADMINISTERING THE MEDICINE

If the child is co-operative (and some are), ask him or her to sit down while the dose is measured out. Then ask him or her to swallow it. Have a favourite drink ready to follow the medicine. If the child takes the medicine without a fuss, always praise him or her.

For the slightly more reluctant child, one carer could sit him or her on their lap and perhaps promise a story afterwards (keep your promise!). The other could then dispense the medicine.

If the child is very reluctant to take the medicine, a firm approach may be needed. The carer should use all his or her powers to encourage the child to take the medicine voluntarily, as there is a risk of the child choking on the medicine if it is given without co-operation.

The child who really cannot be cajoled into taking the medicine may need to be firmly held with one arm around the carer's back and the other in the carer's spare hand. The second carer can then give the medicine when the child opens his or her mouth. There is, of course, one problem with this method, which is that the child might spit the medicine out. (Bribery may come into play here – 'if you take this medicine, you can watch a video for 10 minutes'.)

If the child really finds the flavour unpalatable, it might be necessary to ask the doctor if any other similar preparation is available.

Never pour the dose into a drink, as the child may not finish the drink, it would be impossible to estimate how much of the dose has been taken.

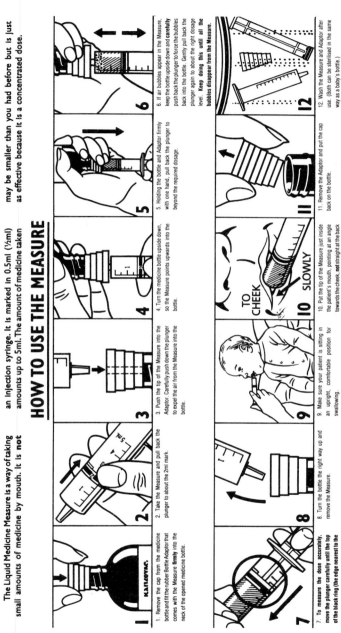

Figure 14   Use of a liquid measure

Eye Drops

The carer washes his or her hands. A young child is best placed on his or her back; the older child may sit with the head extended backwards. Ideally, two adults should be present so that one can hold the child and the other can put the drops in at an opportune time. Care must be taken not to touch the infected eye with the bottle. (See figures 15 and 16.)

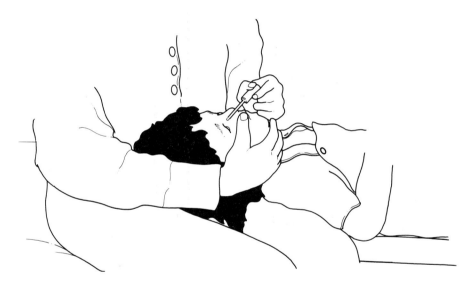

Figure 15   Administration of eye drops (1)   The hands should be washed first. The bottle should be held upside down until a drop forms at the end. The bottle should then be brought across to the child's eye without touching it and the drop released at an opportune time. Ideally, have a distractor behind the child to encourage him or her to look back.

The child will require reassurance during this procedure, because although the instillation of the drops should not be uncomfortable, it is difficult for a young child to keep still in this position for very long.

The person giving the eye drops could place the index finger of one hand just below the lower eyelid and gently pull this down. The other hand holding the dropper should rest on the child's head. The

54

prescribed number of eye drops should then be placed in the space formed between the eye and the lower eyelid. It may be helpful with a co-operative child to play a game such as 'tell me what you can see on the wall behind you' (remember to put a picture there first!). In this way the child is less likely to blink just as the drop is going into the eye.

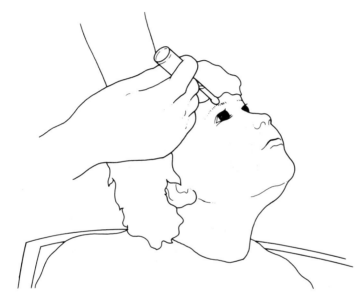

Figure 16   Administration of eye drops (2)   An older child can sit down and hold the head back. The carer can administer the eye drops from behind the child.

It is also a good idea to suggest that he or she tries to count to three before opening the eye. Once the drop has gone into the eye and the child has blinked, some liquid will run out, and this should be gently wiped away with a clean tissue, which should then be discarded.

Ear drops

The carer washes his or her hands. Ideally, two people are needed to instil ear drops into a young child's ear. The child should be placed on his or her back and the head turned so that the affected ear is uppermost (see figure 17). One carer should gently hold the child in this position, while the other rests the hand with the dropper gently on the side of the child's head. The pinna (earlobe) is then held whilst the required number of drops are instilled into the ear. The child is gently held in this position for a few minutes. Once the child holds his or her head up some liquid may escape; this should be wiped away with a clean tissue, which should then be discarded.

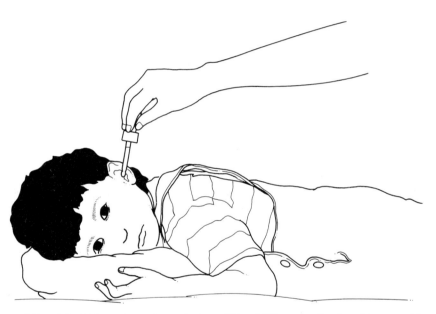

Figure 17   Administration of ear drops   The child turns the head to one side and keeps it to the side for several minutes after administration.

Nose Drops

The carer washes his or her hands. The child should be positioned across the carer's knee with the head extended, as shown in figure 18.

A second carer should then place the dropper close to the nostril and instil the prescribed number of drops. The child should then be kept in this position for approximately one minute.

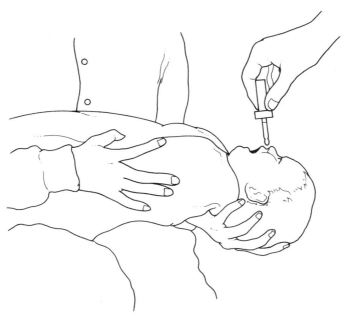

Figure 18   Administration of nose drops   The child should be positioned across the carer's knee with the head extended. A second carer should place the dropper close to the nostril and install the prescribed number of drops.

Topical Medicines (Creams and Ointments)

A cream or ointment may be prescribed for various skin conditions; instructions for application must be followed. Ideally, disposable gloves should be worn when applying topical medicine to protect the carer against absorption of the medication.

Rectal Administration

Very few prescribed medicines in Britain are given rectally. However, sometimes if a child has epilepsy and 'one fit runs into another', a rectal administration of the prescribed medication may be needed. In general, rectal medicines are given by a trained nurse or doctor. However, if a carer is in charge of a child with epilepsy, it may be necessary for the employer to teach him or her the technique.

Injections

The carer may find him or herself looking after a child who requires injections. This skill requires specialist training. If this skill is to be part of the workload, the employer will need to arrange this training with a doctor or nurse.

The Medicine Cabinet

In the day nursery, playgroup, school, etc., there will be a first-aid box. The workplace will have a set policy as to the contents of that box, and the carer should make him or herself familiar with the contents.

In the home, there is often a medicine chest (out of the reach of children), which should be locked and the key kept near at hand (but not actually in the lock). The contents should be checked at regular intervals, and medicines that have passed their use-by date should be discarded.

STUDENT ACTIVITIES

1 Find out the desired and also the unwanted effects of the commonly used medications paracetamol and antibiotics. Make a list that you can keep for easy reference.

2 Find out the policies in your workplace on administration of medicines.

6

THE PROFESSIONALS

The Parents

Although not childcare professionals in the true sense of the word, it is the parents who provide the majority of care for the child and who (almost always) have the child's best interests at heart. They initiate treatment if the child is unwell by nursing him or her and, if necessary, by seeking medical advice. They give the child any medicine and carry out the advice given by the doctor. A carer employed as a nanny may take over many of these duties.

The Primary Health Care Team

When a child is unwell, the carer may need to ask for advice from a health visitor, general practitioner, or perhaps the nurse in the health centre. These professionals, together with the community midwife and the district nurse, make up the **Primary Health Care team**. This team is generally supported by receptionists, and sometimes includes other professionals, such as the school health nurse, the community psychiatric nurse and a social worker. In some areas, there is also a community paediatric nurse attached to the team. These people work together to provide an effective service to clients in the community. The role of the team is not only the care and treatment of people who are unwell, but also health education and health promotion among healthy people. The team may be based in a health-authority-owned health centre or in a privately-owned medical centre (the surgery) or they may be based in separate accommodation. However, whatever the accommodation, they meet on a regular basis to discuss the care of their clients. These regular meetings help to ensure that the clients receive a high standard of care.

THE ROLES OF THE MEMBERS OF THE PRIMARY HEALTH CARE TEAM

General Practitioner

A general practitioner (GP) has trained as a doctor and then completed another three years' training, including a year as a trainee general practitioner. He or she is involved with the promotion of health and the treatment of illness.

When a child's birth is registered, the parents receive a card with a National Health number on it. This is taken along to the surgery, and the child can then be registered with the GP of the parents' choice. In some rural areas, the GP may dispense medicines from the surgery, but in less rural areas, prescriptions need to be taken to the local chemist in order to be dispensed.

Health Visitor

The health visitor is a qualified nurse who has completed a course in health visiting. He or she is involved in the promotion of health and the prevention of ill health.

Within the field of child care, he or she is particularly involved in antenatal care, postnatal care and the care of the pre-school child. He or she, together with the community midwife, often run a parentcraft class in the health centre. The health visitor is involved in visiting the newborn and will subsequently see them in the child health clinics. He or she will be available to offer help and advice on all sorts of matters concerning child care. In particular, he or she may discuss feeding problems, sleep problems, the crying baby and immunisation.

Practice Nurse

The practice nurse is a Registered General Nurse employed by a group of general practitioners (or a single-handed GP) and is responsible for seeing and treating some of the minor conditions. He or she may also be responsible for giving advice in clinics such as the asthma clinic. In this position, the nurse may give routine immunisations to children after they have been seen by the doctor.

Community Midwife

The community midwife works with the doctor to provide antenatal care for pregnant mothers and may be involved in delivering babies in a general practice unit, within the district general hospital or possibly at home. The midwife will be involved in postnatal care, usually until the tenth day after delivery, although in some circumstances this may be extended until twenty-eight days after delivery. The midwife usually works with the health visitor to provide parentcraft classes in the community.

Social Worker

The social worker may have qualified in one of a number of ways, but will have gained the Diploma in Social Work. He or she is employed by the social services department and may be based in a central office with other social workers or in a health centre. Social workers may be appointed to work as Day Care Advisors or may be involved in child protection and various aspects of family support. The social worker takes referrals from many sources, for example the GP, the health visitor, the school nurse, and may also take referrals from clients who feel that they need help and guidance. Social workers are also based in hospitals.

Community Paediatric Nurse

A community paediatric nurse is employed in some districts. Nowadays, children who are unwell are discharged earlier from hospital than in the past. This is partly because it is recognised that children find it less stressful to be cared for at home; once trained in the day-to-day management of their child, parents find it easier to care for the family when they are all under one roof; it also releases a hospital bed for another child. The community paediatric nurse works with the family to enable individual care to be given in the child's own home. He or she will work with other members of the Primary Health Care team in order to organise the care needed. Children who benefit from this type of care include those who have been in hospital for surgery, appendicitis for example, diabetics and sometimes children for whom strict bedrest has been advised. The specialist knowledge of the community paediatric nurse will be required for day-to-day management of the patient, such as a diabetic child who has developed an infection.

School Nurse

The school nurse, employed by the Health Authority, is a Registered General Nurse who may also have a School Nursing Certificate. In many areas, the school health nurse will divide his or her time between several schools and will be responsible for assisting with school medicals, health promotion, health education and care of children with special needs. His or her responsibilities also include advising the school about managing relevant medical problems and ensuring that the school is aware of current policies on the care of certain conditions. He or she may be involved in helping the doctor with medical examinations. Some schools (usually special schools) have a school health nurse in the premises at all times.

The school nurse employed by the Education Authority is not necessarily a qualified nurse. Generally, he or she has a First Aid Certificate. His or her role is to deal with day-to-day problems, such as children falling over and grazing their knees or feeling unwell. The Education Authority school nurse will request medical help if necessary and will liaise with the school nurse (employed by the Health Authority).

The Secondary Health Care Team

In the hospital, there is a wide variety of professionals.

Often, if a child is admitted to a ward, there is a 'Rogue's Gallery' (named photographs of all the staff working on the ward) on the wall as the child enters the ward. These are often necessary, as increasingly professionals are discarding uniforms in an attempt to be less intimidating to the child.

THE ROLES OF MEMBERS OF THE SECONDARY HEALTH TEAM

Nurses

There are usually many different nurses on the ward; some are qualified, some are in training to be Registered Sick Children's Nurses, some may be training to be Registered General Nurses and some may be Auxiliary Nurses. It is recommended that eighty per cent of nurses working on a paediatric ward should be Registered Sick Children's Nurses.

At any one time, a specific nurse (the 'named nurse') will be assigned to a child and this nurse will be responsible for the care of the child during his or her time on duty. Generally, he or she will have several children in their care and will usually work with parents or other carers to plan and implement the child's care during his or her span of duty. In some hospitals, the same nurse will be allocated to the child for several days at a time to allow continuity of care. This does have the effect of reducing the number of people to whom the child has to relate. However, in a twenty-four-hour period, the child will need to go to know at least two nurses. Some hospitals operate a twelve-hour shift system and some an eight-hour shift system.

Doctors

During a stay in hospital, the child may meet many different grades of doctors. The **senior house officer** (SHO) is the doctor that the child will see most often. He or she will have completed five years in medical school and will also have worked as a house officer for a year.

The **registrar** is senior to the SHO, having worked as an SHO for several years. He or she either has an additional qualification in paediatrics or is working towards one.

The **senior registrar** (SR) is, as the name implies, more senior than the registrar and is gaining further experience whilst waiting for final promotion to the position of consultant. The SR may be involved in research as well as working on the wards.

The **consultant** specialising in sick children is called a paediatrician. He or she has ultimate responsibility for the patients. The paediatric consultant will usually work in the hospital, but may do home visits if requested.

Other Professionals

There may be occasions when the child is referred to other professionals for specialist advice. These may include:

The surgeon
This is a doctor who performs operations, for example if a child has appendicitis.

The radiologist
The child may need some tests before a diagnosis can be made. The radiographer (see below) is the technician who takes X-rays, and the radiologist is the doctor who interprets them. Radiologists also use radiotherapy in the treatment of some conditions, including cancer.

The radiographer
Radiographers have to complete a three-year course and will probably be seen most often when taking X-rays. However, they are also involved in other specialist tests, such as ultrasound tests, which are becoming increasingly common.

The anaesthetist
If a child requires surgery, he or she may need an anaesthetic, and this will be administered by the anaesthetist.

The physiotherapist
The physiotherapist also has to complete a three-year course and may be involved in treatment in a number of ways. He or she has experience in treating people with exercise, manipulation, heat, massage or electrical stimulation (such as ultrasound treatment). The physiotherapist is also involved with the care of people with respiratory conditions, such as cystic fibrosis, asthma and bronchitis.

The play specialist
These people are usually qualified nursery nurses who have had a substantial amount of experience of working with children and may also have completed a one-year hospital play specialist course. His or her role is to encourage children in hospital to play, thus helping them to come to terms with hospitalisation and also to accept their condition. Many hospitals now employ a play specialist for each children's ward, and they are a very important member of the team.

The play therapist
Some hospitals employ a play therapist. He or she has completed a further period of training and usually works with children who have experienced particularly traumatic situations.

The occupational therapist
An occupational therapist will have had three years' training. He or she works mainly with children who have suffered a severe injury or who have a disability and helps them to become as independent as possible. Sometimes, occupational therapists may also be asked to work with children who are considered to be clumsy. Sometimes his or her work will involve the use of special equipment, and he or she will give advice on any alterations which may be needed to the patient's home. The occupational therapist will usually be based in the hospital but will visit the home as and when necessary.

The speech therapist

A speech therapist has to complete three years' training. He or she is involved with how the child communicates, which includes receiving communication as well as self-expression. The speech therapist works in the hospital and in the community.

The dietician

These professionals give advice on the importance of a healthy diet. However, their involvement with the care of children lies in the specific advice necessary for children with, for example, diabetes, food intolerance or a food allergy. Dieticians usually work both in the hospital and in the community. Training takes three years.

The teacher

Many hospitals have schoolrooms and employ trained teachers. It is particularly important for children who are going to be in hospital for a long time not to miss out on their education.

Non-Hospital-Based Professionals

Other non-hospital-based professionals involved with the care of sick children include the following.

CHILD AND FAMILY PSYCHIATRIC SERVICE

This service is community based and is run by a team of professionals headed by a psychiatrist and including a social worker and community psychiatric nurses. Children can be referred to this clinic by a GP or a health visitor, or the family can refer themselves.

A community psychiatric nurse is involved in the assessment and treatment of children (and their families) with mental health problems.

THE COMMUNITY CLINIC

In some areas, GPs do not carry out their own child health surveillance. When this is the case, a clinical medical officer will see the children in a community-based clinic. The clinical medical officer is a qualified doctor who has had extra training in paediatrics. Clinical medical officers may also be seen in specialist clinics.

SCHOOLS

Teachers will usually have trained for three or four years. Obviously the prime responsibility is to educate the children in their care; however, it may well be the teacher who notices the initial signs and symptoms of illness and alerts the parents to the situation.

THE EDUCATIONAL PSYCHOLOGIST

The educational psychologist will have a psychology degree and a teaching qualification and will have undergone further training. A child may be referred to him or her for assessment by the school.

Conclusion

The child may well be overwhelmed by the number of different professionals encountered during the course of an illness. However, it must be stated that only a proportion of ill children are admitted to hospital, and only a proportion of those will meet all the people mentioned above.

STUDENT ACTIVITY

You cannot predict when or if a child will be unwell. However, it is accepted that if the child is prepared in some way, they tend to come to terms with the situation more easily. You are working in a playgroup and have decided to make the theme for the next few weeks 'going to the doctor'.

1   Develop this theme with one or two peers. You could perhaps draw a spider diagram of your ideas.

2   You might like to make a Rogue's Gallery of the people working in the surgeries that the children go to when they are unwell.

3   Invite one or two of the professionals to the playgroup to talk about their role. They might like to take the opportunity to do some health education with the children.

4   Go to the local library and borrow some books that are relevant to your topic. The children's librarian is often very helpful when groups are doing topic work.

5   Back up the topic with plenty of relevant toys, such as the Fisher Price doctor's set and Playmobil hospital. If your group does not have enough money to buy the toys, find out whether you can get access to a toy library.

6   Perhaps you could turn the home corner into a doctor's surgery.

7   The children could be involved in plenty of creative work during this topic: for example, they could paint pictures of themselves feeling unwell.

8   As most children have had some experience of feeling unwell, they are often happy to talk about it, and there is scope for lots of language work.

9   Develop any other thoughts you may have for the topic.

7

FAILURE TO THRIVE

—

'Failure to thrive' is a term used when a child does not conform to the usual pattern of weight gain and growth.

Weight Gain and Growth

Babies are routinely weighed at regular intervals during the first years of life. This weight measurement is the most commonly used measurement of growth. In the first year of life, there is rapid growth, and usually a baby doubles its birth weight by six months and triples it by the age of one year. Whenever a baby is weighed in the clinic, the weight will be plotted on the growth (centile) chart by the health visitor.

GROWTH CHARTS

The latest growth charts (published in 1994) reflect the fact that children in many countries have become taller and heavier at all ages and that they mature earlier and therefore reach their final height at a younger age. This is probably due to improved nutrition and living conditions.

The growth chart has a number of curves printed across it (see figure 19). These curves are percentile (usually called centile) curves. They represent the normal pattern of child weight, height gain and head circumference.

Weight

Most babies will tend to gain weight along the curve from which they started. A child whose weight falls below the 0.4th centile or above the

99.6th centile will be referred to a specialist. Children whose weight starts to cross centiles will also be carefully monitored and referred to a specialist if necessary. This is an indicator that the child may be failing to thrive. Genetic and ethnic factors do need to be taken into account; for instance, Chinese babies tend to be small and therefore lighter.

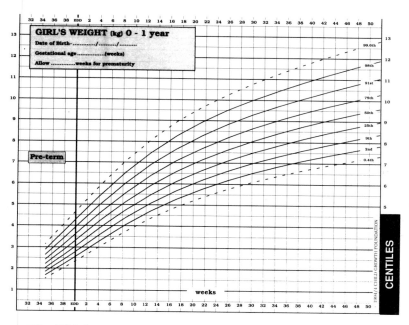

Figure 19   Weight growth chart © Child Growth Foundation

Height

Until the age of two years, the length (i.e. the height) of the baby is measured lying down. The first proper height measurement is made at the age of three years or when the child is sufficiently cooperative for accurate measurement.

Again, children who fall below the 0.4th centile or above the 99.6th centile will be referred to a specialist. Children whose height starts to cross centiles will also be carefully monitored and referred to a specialist if necessary. Children who are either very short or very tall may be at a psychological disadvantage among both adults and peers.

Head Circumference

Measurements of head circumference are made and plotted on the appropriate chart. Babies with a head circumference below the 0.4th centile or above the 99.6th centile will be referred to a specialist. A baby or child with a rapidly growing head will be referred to a paediatrician, as this may be an indication of hydrocephalus. Children whose head circumference starts to cross centiles will be carefully monitored and referred to a specialist if necessary.

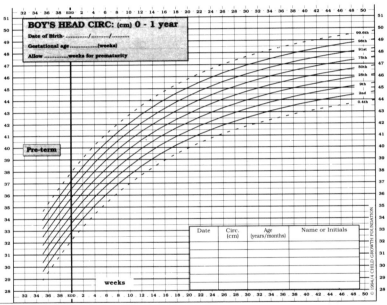

Figure 20   Head circumference growth chart © Child Growth Foundation

Measurements

These are usually carried out by professionals who have been trained to measure accurately. However, the carer should be familiar with the charts and have an understanding of their meaning.

Reasons for failure to thrive

If a baby appears to be failing to thrive, the health visitor will usually explore the issues of feeding with the parents in the first instance, as this is the most likely reason for the problem. However, if this proves not to be the case, other avenues are explored. Problems of weight loss or failure to gain weight are easily recognised if the child attends the child surveillance clinic regularly, because a written record of the child's weight is made and plotted on a growth chart. The health visitor will encourage all parents or carers to attend the clinic regularly, particularly if there is any cause for worry. In a recently weaned baby, failure to thrive is most commonly due to intolerance of a newly introduced food. Weight gain – and thus thriving – will occur if the food is removed from the diet. This is usually a temporary measure, and the food may be re-introduced at a later stage when it will perhaps be tolerated.

Diagnosis of failure to thrive is made initially by the doctor or health visitor in the clinic. The child may then need investigation, which might require hospitalisation.

A child who is failing to thrive may lose weight or fail to gain weight. This may be due to any of a number of the following:

- poor nutritional intake;
- illness and congenital abnormalities not accounted for by poor nutrition;
- poverty;
- child abuse, including neglect;
- hormonal deficiency;
- developmental delay.

POOR NUTRITIONAL INTAKE

Causes of poor nutritional intake include:

- problems associated with feeding;
- breathing difficulties;
- vomiting;
- malabsorption of food.

Problems Associated with Feeding

Usually the health visitor will discuss the possibilities with the carer at length and steps will be taken to rectify obvious misunderstandings such as making up a bottle feed incorrectly. If, however, the problem is less easily identified, it may take all the skills of the health visitor to try to identify the problem, and if he or she is not successful, the child will

71

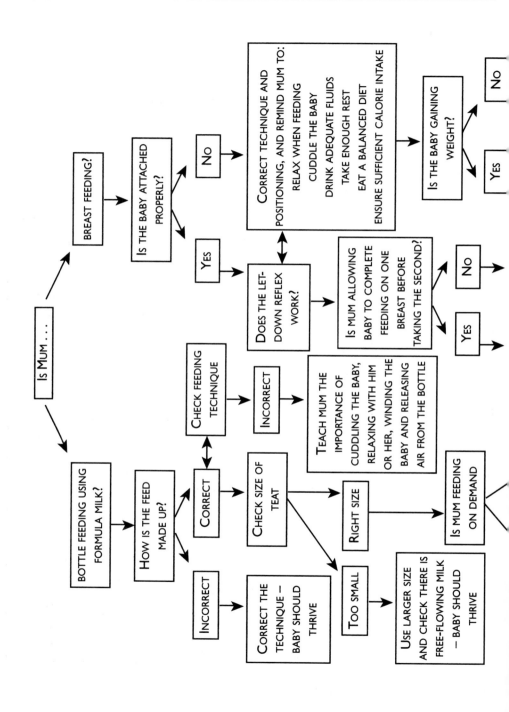

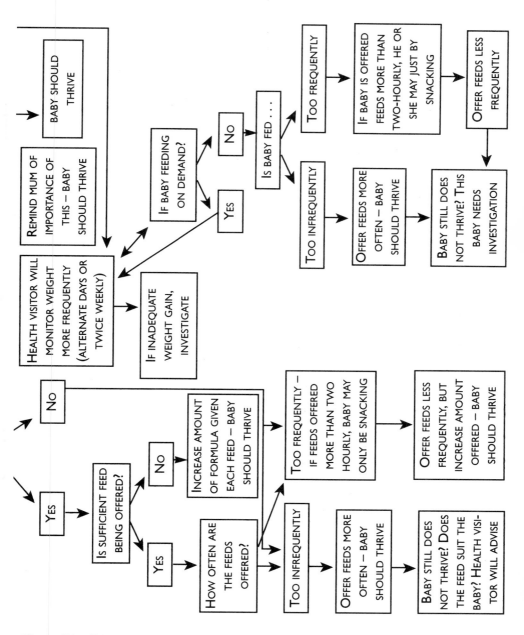

Figure 21   Diagnosis of nutritional problems in babies

need further investigation. (See figure 21 for a guide to diagnosing potential nutritional problems.) The baby may have difficulty with sucking because of breathing difficulties (see below), a cleft palate (which can often be overcome prior to surgery by the use of a specially designed teat or nipple shield) or because of the lack of sucking reflex (some babies born prematurely may not have a very good sucking reflex).

Breathing Difficulties

Breathing problems may make it difficult for a baby to suck adequately. He or she needs to be able to breathe through the nostrils while sucking. The common cold can cause temporary blockage, and the general practitioner may, in some circumstances, prescribe nose drops to be used as directed until the blockage has resolved. (This is only a temporary cause for failure to thrive.)

Vomiting

A child who is vomiting frequently over a period of time is unlikely to thrive. Reasons for vomiting include:

Pyloric stenosis
This is a congenital abnormality in which the pyloric sphincter (the muscle controlling the point where the duodenum and stomach join) is thickened and narrowed. The undigested milk cannot all pass through, and projectile vomiting results. This condition usually presents itself early in the child's life and can be corrected by surgery.

Hiatus hernia
This is due to a weakness in the diaphragm which results in a portion of the stomach being pulled up into the thoracic (chest) cavity. The cardiac sphincter (the muscle controlling the point where the oesophagus and stomach join) is therefore not working effectively, and the stomach contents flow back into the oesophagus (gullet). This condition can usually be corrected by surgery.

Gastroenteritis
This is an infection of the gastro-intestinal tract which results in diarrhoea and or vomiting. It is highly infectious.

Whooping cough
This is an infectious disease in which the paroxysms of coughing may

result in the child vomiting. If this occurs, it is important to offer them another feed.

Malabsorption of Food

Any child who is not adequately absorbing food will fail to thrive. This condition tends to become apparent after weaning.

Coeliac disease

This condition is due to an intolerance to gluten (a protein found in wheat and some other cereals). Gluten has the effect of flattening the villi (the finger-like projections found in the small intestine), thus impairing absorption of food. The child will fail to thrive and will often be miserable. He or she may have a distended abdomen and pass frequent, foul-smelling stools. Once the condition has been diagnosed and the gluten has been removed from the diet, the child will thrive again.

Phenylketonuria (PKU)

This is a hereditary condition, usually diagnosed by the Guthrie test (a sample of blood is taken from the child via a heel prick) which is routinely done on the fifth day after birth. In this condition, the child is intolerant to phenylalanine (an amino acid which is a basic unit of protein). Treatment involves the elimination of almost all the phenylalanine from the diet to prevent mental handicap developing. Treatment must commence within the first weeks of life.

Galactosaemia

This is a familial disease which is caused by an inability to absorb galactose (a nutrient found in milk). It can lead to mental handicap, cirrhosis of the liver and cataracts. After diagnosis, a dietician will advise the family, as treatment involves giving a diet free of galactose or lactose. This condition may be identified by taking a sample of blood from the umbilical cord or by doing a urine test. These tests will be carried out on all babies where there is a family history of galactosaemia.

Of course, failure to thrive may simply be the result of the child receiving an inadequately balanced diet. If the child thrived prior to being weaned, the health visitor should find out about the diet the child is receiving and may need to discuss with the parent(s) the importance of a balanced diet.

ILLNESS

Children may fail to thrive if suffering from long-term illnesses, including the following.

Cystic fibrosis

This is an inherited disease. Secretions in the body are thicker than usual, with the most commonly affected organs being the lungs and the pancreas. In the lungs, the thick, sticky mucus blocks the air tubes, with the result that the child may suffer from repeated chest infections and have difficulty in breathing at times. The thick secretions in the pancreas result in digestive enzymes being unable to reach the digestive tract, thus impairing the digestion of food. The child therefore fails to thrive. Treatment involves giving pancreatic enzymes by mouth in an enteric (protective) coated form so that they are not attacked by the acidity in the stomach, and teaching the parents to give chest physiotherapy on a daily basis.

Cerebral Palsy

This is a condition in which part of the child's brain does not function correctly or has not developed normally. This usually results in muscle control and movement being affected. Some of these children also fail to thrive.

Asthma

This is a disease of the lungs. There is increased sensitivity of the air tubes which causes them to swell and thus become narrowed. There is also an increase in mucus production. Many children who have chronic asthma may have slightly stunted growth.

Urinary tract infections

These are fairly common in young children and may be a cause of failure to thrive where diagnosis of the infection has not been made.

Heart disease

This is seen in approximately eight out of every 1000 births. In infants with large defects, the child may fail to thrive; this is partly due to the fact that they are often breathless because of the less effective heart and tend to suffer from repeated chest infections.

POVERTY

An inadequate income may lead to an inadequate diet, which will inevitably have an effect on the child and his or her ability to thrive. The health visitor will be the key worker and may invite a social worker to visit the family to help them claim for any benefits to which they may be entitled. (Involvement of the social worker in such cases requires consent from the family concerned.)

Poverty can lead to stress within the family, and stress can and often does have a negative effect on the child. Family stress may lead to a lack of stimulation for the child and subsequent developmental delay. In extreme cases, family stress can lead to non-accidental injury of the child.

CHILD ABUSE AND NEGLECT

The term 'child abuse' may include physical abuse, emotional abuse, neglect or sexual abuse.

Physical Abuse

The child may be physically injured, or the injury not prevented, by a carer. This form of abuse may also include giving a child poisonous substances (alcohol, inappropriate drugs, etc.) or attempting to suffocate or drown the child. Children who are physically abused may also be nutritionally and emotionally neglected. Failure to thrive and developmental delay may be the presenting factors in the child clinic.

Emotional Abuse

The child is psychologically ill-treated, which, in time, affects his or her behaviour and development. The carer of an emotionally abused child will continuously fail to show the child affection and love or will shout, bully, reject or threaten the child so that he or she loses self-confidence and self-esteem. The ill-treatment may lead to failure to thrive.

Neglect

The child may have been persistently or severely deprived of essential needs. There are numerous reasons why parents may neglect their children: for example, if the baby is unwanted, if the parents have not established a good bond with the child or if the mother is suffering from depression or mental illness. The first sign of neglect in these children is that they often fail to thrive.

Sexual Abuse

The child is forced to take part in sexual activities which may include intercourse, masturbation, fondling or exposure to pornography. These acts may lead to unhappiness and to failure to thrive.

These causes of failure to thrive can occur at any time in the child's life, but are most commonly seen in the first five years, with the majority of cases being seen in children under the age of one. The child's weight will fall away from the expected centile curve. The child may be disinterested in eating (although he or she will usually eat readily when in hospital) and may appear to have lost interest in activities previously enjoyed – he or she may appear to be a rather sad child. Once these children have been identified, they may be put on the child protection register so that they are then regularly followed up.

Children may be abused because parents/carers:

- do not meet the needs of the child;
- do not protect the child;
- harm the child.

Recognising Abuse – The Role of the Carer

Each area in the UK has a child protection committee. Through this committee, procedures have been established.

If a carer suspects that a child has been abused, this suspicion must be reported. If the carer is working in a junior position, the suspicion may be initially discussed with someone in a more senior position. It will then need to be reported to the social services department, police or NSPCC. The carer should write down his or her observations and include the date and time, a drawing of any injuries and notes and records of what is said. The child is protected by the Children Act 1989.

This section on child abuse is not a comprehensive guide for carers, but merely serves as an introduction. The carer is advised to attend a course on child abuse. Social services often organise the courses. The local library will be able to obtain books on the subjects. Ensure that you are familiar with the Children Act.

HORMONAL DEFICIENCY

Hormonal deficiency is uncommon in childhood; however, when there is a deficiency such as with hypothyroidism, there may be an effect on intellectual and physical growth.

Hypothyroidism

Hypothyroidism is caused by an under secretion of the hormone Thyroxine which is produced in the thyroid gland. This is usually screened for at the same time the Guthrie test is carried out (five days after birth). If for some reason this test has not been carried out or if the child has developed hypothyroidism at a later stage, it may become apparent because of slowing in growth.

Growth Hormone Deficiency

Some children have delayed growth because of a deficiency of growth hormone. Once this has been diagnosed, affected children may have regular injections of growth hormone.

DEVELOPMENTAL DELAY

Developmental delay is often not apparent until later in the child's first year. Of these children, some simply show an unexplained failure to thrive.

Conclusion

'Failure to thrive' is a term used to describe many diagnoses. However, it is a problem which can often be identified by the various health care professionals during the child surveillance at the health clinic, and, once investigated, appropriate treatment can be initiated. Frequently, it is the parent who will bring the child to the doctor because he or she may have noticed that the child is not gaining weight as he or she should be. The nursery nurse may also observe a child who is apparently failing to thrive and would need to discuss this first with the parents (if working as a nanny). However, if he or she is working with children in another setting, any worries would need to be discussed with the supervisor first.

STUDENT ACTIVITY

1   'Children who are either very short or very tall may be at a psychological disadvantage from adults and peers.'

   Discuss this statement in a group, with particular reference to:
   - the expectations of a short/tall child with respect to age;
   - the 'mothering' of a short child;
   - the difficulties of the tall child when engaging in physical play with peers.

2   You have been asked to demonstrate 'how to make up a bottle feed' to mothers-to-be at a parentcraft class. List the equipment you will need. Which formulas will you take along for demonstration purposes? Give your reasons.

   You will need to stress the importance of making the feed up according to the manufacturer's instructions. How do you plan to emphasise the importance of this?

   You may have the chance to evaluate your session. Plan a written evaluation form that may be used.

8

CAUSES OF INFECTION

—

This chapter deals with the causes, spread and prevention of infection. It also covers the body's defences against infection.

Infection occurs when an organism enters the body and causes a harmful reaction. Microscopic organisms capable of causing infection are called **pathogens**. Not all micro-organisms are pathogens; for instance, bacteria that live in the large intestine provide a source of vitamins.

Pathogens

There are three main groups of pathogens: bacteria, viruses and fungi.

BACTERIA

These are single-celled micro-organisms. They are capable of rapid reproduction in the right conditions. An example of a bacterium is salmonella, which can cause food poisoning. Their growth is inhibited by sunlight and by antibiotics.

VIRUSES

These are smaller than bacteria. They can only grow when they have gained access into a living cell. Examples of viruses are the common cold and Human Immunodeficiency Virus (HIV).

FUNGI

These are usually larger than bacteria and may be multicellular. Ringworm is caused by a fungi.

Other organisms that can cause infection (and are not microscopic) include roundworms (for example, threadworms), flatworms (for example, tapeworms) and insects (for example, head lice).

ENTRY OF PATHOGENS

Pathogens may be:

- inhaled – for example, the common cold virus;
- ingested (eaten) – for example, salmonella;
- inoculated (introduced via the skin) – for example, organisms that cause wound infections.

Spread of Infection

Infection may be spread directly, for example by kissing or by sexual contact, or indirectly. Indirect spread includes air, food, drink, soil or fomites (objects that have been contaminated by an infected person and are then used by another person, for example crockery or cutlery).

Defences against Infection

The body has several methods of defence against infection from pathogens.

- The skin acts in two ways: its intact surface is a mechanical barrier, and the secretions it produces provide a hostile medium to pathogens.
- Mucous membranes line all the internal surfaces of the body. The mucus traps pathogens, and they are then removed from the body. For example, in the respiratory tract there are cilia (tiny hair-like projections) that waft the mucus to the outside.
- Lyzozyme is an antibacterial enzyme found in tears, saliva and urine, thus giving defence to the eye, mouth and bladder.
- The acid medium found in the stomach kills off many pathogens.
- Breast-fed babies harbour non-pathogenic bacteria in their gut which produce an acid to help protect against gut infections.

Sometimes, despite these defences, the infective organism gains entry to the body. When this occurs, there is an **inflammatory response**, which may be apparent as the area becomes inflamed, hot, red and uncomfortable. This response results in many blood cells coming into contact with the pathogens. The white blood cells will then attempt to destroy them.

The inflammatory response may be followed by the **specific defence response** mounted by the lymphatic system. The lymphatic system is made up of lymphoid tissue interconnected by lymph vessels. The lymph nodes (see page 33) are widely distributed to cope with the various possible entry points of micro-organisms. Lymphocytes are produced in this system and they are the active force. There are two main types of lymphocytes: the B-lymphocyte and the T-lymphocyte.

The B-lymphocytes are involved in the production of antibodies which attack the pathogen, thereby defending the body against illness. The T-lymphocytes multiply in the presence of pathogens. They attach themselves to cells that have been invaded by the pathogens and release chemicals to aid their destruction.

When the pathogens have been defeated, the child will regain health. A small number of antibodies remain in circulation, thus providing protection against further invasion from that particular pathogen.

IMMUNISATION

Immunisation methods have been developed to help strengthen the body's defences. (Immunisation schedules are on page 25.) Immunisation can be given actively or passively.

Passive Immunisation

Serum (the fluid part of the blood that is left when the blood cells have been removed) containing the antibodies is given to people because either they are not manufacturing enough antibodies themselves or they are at high risk from an infection (for example, a child receiving chemotherapy (see page 167) who comes into contact with an infectious disease may receive passive immunity). Passive immunity is short lived.

Note: the foetus acquires passive immunity from the mother, and this helps to protect the baby from infection in the first months of life. It is further 'topped up' if the mother breast feeds, as antibodies are given to the baby via the breast milk.

Active Immunisation

Here, the person is given an 'inactivated' (harmless) form of the pathogen or modified form of the toxin (the poisonous substance produced by the pathogen) called a toxoid which will provoke the immune response and the production of antibodies. These methods do not cause the disease. Since the body itself has produced these antibodies, the immunity lasts considerably longer than with passive immunity.

Prevention of Infection

It is important that the carer is aware of his or her role in the prevention of infection. A child is more susceptible to infection than an adult because:

- the immune response is not fully developed;
- his or her play often involves being in close proximity to other children who may have infections;
- children need to be taught and reminded about acceptable standards of hygiene – children will often follow the example set by their carers, and these examples must therefore be of a high standard;
- many young children often put their hands in their mouths, which means that they transmit infection from their hands;
- children tend to fall more often than adults, and therefore cuts and grazes are more common.

The two main ways of preventing infection are reducing susceptibility to infection and controlling pathogens.

REDUCING SUSCEPTIBILITY TO INFECTION

This can be achieved by:

- maintaining a good standard of health (which includes eating a well-balanced diet, taking regular exercise, having adequate rest and sleep, avoiding stress, not inhaling cigarette smoke);
- keeping a high standard of personal hygiene (which includes washing the body, hair and clothes regularly);

- maintaining an intact skin by avoiding cuts and using moisturisers if the skin is dry (dry skin may crack and infection may be introduced) – any cuts should be covered with waterproof dressing during waking hours;
- ensuring the child's and the carers' immunisations are up to date.

CONTROLLING PATHOGENS

There are several methods of reducing pathogens which may be used, although the carer will probably only use only one or two methods in the workplace.

- Chemical sterilisation is one method. This can be achieved by means of liquid, crystals or a sterilising tablet which is added to water in recommended quantity to produce a sterilising solution. This method is often used to sterilise babies' bottles. It is important that they are thoroughly clean before being immersed and that they stay immersed for the recommended time.
- Boiling has a similar effect. Equipment can be completely immersed in boiling water for five minutes, thus killing off pathogens.
- Use of a steam steriliser is another method. These units can be purchased and are effective at destroying pathogens when the manufacturer's instructions are followed carefully.
- The number of pathogens in the environment can be reduced by good ventilation.

Checklist for Limiting Infection

The following list outlines many ways of limiting the spread of infection.

- Ensure a high standard of personal hygiene is maintained, which includes using a good hand-washing technique. Many people wash their hands without washing the tips of their fingers, and many miss areas on the hands. Hands should be washed after any 'dirty' job, for example dusting, hoovering or gardening.
- Children should be taught to wash their hands after using the toilet, before meals and after messy play.

- Hands should be dried using disposable paper towels, individual personal towels or by using automatic hand driers.
- Maintain a high level of hygiene in the home and the workplace. Surfaces should be cleaned regularly during the day, particularly before and after meals.
- Toys need to be kept clean.
- Toilets, basins and baths should be cleaned regularly.
- Food should be stored in a clean refrigerator; uncooked meats should be stored on the bottom shelf, preferably on a plate so that dripping juices cannot contaminate other food. Cooked meats should be kept on the top shelves, away from uncooked meats.
- Food should be thoroughly cooked.
- Food should not be eaten after the use-by date.
- Food can be reheated, but care must be taken to heat it thoroughly.
- Food should be protected from flies.
- Babies' bottles (and dummies) should be sterilised before use until they no longer contain milk.
- Animals should not be allowed in the kitchen.
- Animal excreta in the garden should be disposed of in a place which is inaccessible to all children.
- Care should be taken when dealing with cat-litter trays. They need to be left where they are inaccessible to children.
- Cats and dogs should be regularly wormed.
- Kitchen sinks must be thoroughly cleaned on a regular basis.
- Dishcloths and tea towels should be washed daily.
- Good washing and washing-up techniques should be practised.
- The mouth and nose should be covered when coughing and sneezing, and the hands washed afterwards.
- Noses should be wiped with paper tissues, and these should be disposed of by flushing them down the toilet.
- Carpets should be vacuumed regularly.
- Floors should be washed regularly.
- The carer should stay away from work when he or she is unwell.
- The carer should educate children about hygiene and encourage cleanliness.
- Sometimes it may be necessary to suggest that a child should be cared for at home when he or she is unwell; for example, the child with a heavy cold would feel happier and more secure in his or her own home, where there is little chance of infecting other children.

STUDENT ACTIVITIES

1 You are advertising for a cleaner to clean the day nursery where you are in charge.

- Write a list of tasks that you would expect him or her to do.
- Beside each task, give an explanation of the importance of this activity in helping to maintain a healthy environment for the children and the staff.
- Prepare an induction session of two hours for the new cleaner. You will need to show him or her around the nursery, but will need to stress the methods you expect him or her to use when cleaning.

2 Wash your hands in the usual way, but note any areas not adequately washed. Change the technique so that it is more effective.

Now observe school-aged children washing their hands and plan a short (no more than a few minutes) teaching session demonstrating a good hand-washing technique. Follow this up by observing the children who were present at the teaching session again to see if your advice has been adopted. It may take several attempts before change is seen in all the children.

3 Children admitted to hospital with an infectious disease may need to be 'barrier nursed'. Find out what this means and list the special precautions that are required.

9

CHILDHOOD INFECTIONS – SPECIFIC CARE AND TREATMENT

This chapter is intended for use as a reference section on childhood infections. The information can be accessed easily, as it is grouped according to the area of the body affected: for example, conjunctivitis is found in the section on infections of the eye.

Babies are, to some extent, protected against infection in the first few months of life because they usually have immunity in the form of antibodies, passed from their mothers whilst *in utero* (see page 83). This immunity may be further boosted by the antibodies that are passed through the breast milk if the baby is breast fed. The immunity from these antibodies is relatively short lived, and in time the baby will manufacture his or her own antibodies in response to infections.

General Points

- Only specific care is included in this section. For general care of the sick child, refer to page 39.
- In many of the conditions in this chapter, the child will have a raised temperature. Refer to page 46 for information on reducing the temperature.
- If you are worried about the child at any time, ask for advice from the health visitor or the doctor.
- Children can resume their usual social activities, including school or playgroup, etc., only when they are well.

Common Infectious Diseases

CHICKEN-POX (VIRAL)

incubation period
13–21 days

time child is infectious
from one day before the rash until scabs have dried

Characteristics

A child with chicken-pox:

- may be 'off colour' for a few days before the appearance of the rash;
- may have a raised temperature and a headache;
- will have a rash which starts on the head and behind the ears. This rash eventually covers the whole body. It is characterised by red spots, blisters and dry scabs all being present at one time once the infection has established itself. The rash is itchy.

Specific Care

- Keep the child's nails short so that he or she cannot tear the skin when scratching.
- Keep the child cool and use calamine lotion dabbed on the skin to reduce itching. Sometimes medication to prevent itching may need to be prescribed.

Complications

Chicken-pox usually passes without complications. However, scratching spots may cause them to be infected and result in scaring. Chest infections and rarely encephalitis (inflammation of the brain) may occur.

MUMPS (VIRAL)

incubation period
17–21 days

time child is infectious
seven days before swelling and up to nine days after

This is a condition where the virus affects the salivary glands, particularly the parotid glands which are found below the ears.

Characteristics

The child:

- will be 'off colour' for a few days before the more obvious features of mumps become apparent;
- may have a raised temperature (which may last up to a week);
- may have a headache;
- will have one or both parotid glands swollen, causing discomfort;
- will have a dry mouth;
- may encounter pain when eating and drinking.

Specific Care

- Paracetamol will help to relieve the pain and reduce the temperature.
- The child should be encouraged to have plenty to drink.
- The child may find sloppy foods easier to eat.

Complications

This is usually a mild disease; however, the child may develop mumps meningitis (inflammation of the lining of the brain) or encephalitis (inflammation of the brain). The testes may swell in a boy, and the ovaries may swell in a girl, both causing pain locally.

RUBELLA (GERMAN MEASLES) (VIRAL)

incubation period   **time child is infectious**
14–21 days   from a few days before the rash until four days later

Characteristics

The child:

- has a rash of small, pink spots (lasting two to three days) and swollen lymph glands at the back of the neck and often elsewhere;
- may be a little 'off colour' for a few days before the rash and may have a slight fever.

Specific Care

As rubella is usually mild, there is no specific care. However, rubella caught in the first few months of pregnancy can seriously damage an unborn child, causing deafness, blindness, mental retardation and malformations of the heart. Unfortunately, it is infectious for seven days before the rash is apparent, and it is therefore important to inform women of child-bearing age who have been in contact with an infectious child.

Rubella immunisation was introduced for all girls in the UK in 1970. In 1988, it was introduced in the form of MMR (measles, mumps and rubella), and both boys and girls are offered immunisation at thirteen months.

Complications

There is a slight risk of encephalitis (inflammation of the brain).

MEASLES (VIRAL)

incubation period
10–14 days

time child is infectious
from one day before first symptom until four days later

This is an unpleasant and very infectious viral childhood disease.

Characteristics

The child:

- is unwell for three or four days before the rash appears;
- will have Koplick's spots (small, white spots) on the inside of the cheeks before the skin rash is apparent;
- will often have a temperature, a runny nose, red eyes and a cough;
- will have a rash, behind the ears and at the back of the neck initially, which then spreads all over the body – the rash is reddish-brown in colour, the spots are flat and joined together and look blotchy.
- will often dislike bright light.

Specific Care

- Control of the child's temperature is important, as it may rise to 40°C.
- Ensure that the child has plenty of fluids.
- The child will be comfortable if cared for in a darkened room.

Complications

The child may develop conjunctivitis, otitis media (inflammation of the middle ear), chest infections or encephalitis (inflammation of the brain).

WHOOPING COUGH (PERTUSSIS) (BACTERIAL)

incubation period
7–10 days

time child is infectious
from seven days after exposure until twenty-one days later

Whooping cough is a serious bacterial disease; babies under the age of one are most at risk.

Characteristics

The child:

- will have a cold and cough initially;
- later there may be prolonged bouts of coughing, during which the child may have difficulty in breathing;
- may go blue at this stage due to lack of oxygen;
- will probably make a characteristic whoop at the end of the bout of coughing;
- may also vomit at this stage;
- will have a cough which may last several weeks.

Specific Care

- Antibiotics should be given as early as possible to reduce the severity of the disease.
- The child should be cared for in a smoke-free atmosphere.
- During a coughing bout, the child should be sat upright.
- The carer should reassure the child during an attack – any panic in the carer may be frightening for the child.
- The child should sleep in the same room as the parents, who will need a lot of patience as the child will be unwell for several weeks.
- The child will need plenty of rest, as the bouts of coughing will disturb his or her sleep.
- After vomiting, the older child will need a mouth rinse. A baby should be offered another feed.

- Severe cases of whooping cough are admitted to hospital where they are barrier nursed and specific care given.
- A doctor should be called if the child's condition deteriorates or if there is any difficulty in breathing.

Complications

The vomiting may lead to loss of weight, malnutrition and dehydration. The child is at risk from many other complications, including pneumonia and bronchitis, which may lead to permanent lung damage, and a hernia because of the severe coughing. Lack of oxygen during a bout of coughing may lead to convulsions. Encephalitis (inflammation of the brain) may occur. Babies under the age of six months are particularly prone to complications and may die as a result of whooping cough.

Infections of the Nervous System

MENINGITIS

Meningitis is an inflammation of the meninges (protective coverings of the brain and spinal cord). It is a serious and potentially fatal disease. Meningitis affects children more commonly than adults.

Cause

Meningitis can be caused by bacteria (usually meningococcus, pneumococcus or haemophilis influenza) and viruses. The viral form of the disease is usually less serious.

Characteristics

The child:

- may become very unwell, very quickly;
- will usually have a raised temperature;
- will usually have a headache;
- may be nauseated or actually vomit;
- may dislike bright light (photophobia);
- may have a stiff neck;
- may become drowsy;

- may have a rash and bruising.

In a baby, it can be more difficult to diagnose, but the following characteristics should be looked for. The baby:

- will often have a high-pitched cry;
- may refuse feeds;
- will be very irritable;
- may have bulging of the fontanelles;
- may have a convulsion.

Specific Care

- If meningitis is suspected, medical help should be sought without delay.
- If the child is very unwell, he or she should be taken to the accident and emergency department at the nearest hospital.
- The child's temperature should be reduced to prevent a convulsion (see page 48).
- Darken the child's room.
- Reassure the child and stay calm.

A child with meningitis will be admitted to hospital, where he or she will be barrier nursed to prevent the spread of infection. The GP may give antibiotics to the child before he or she is transferred to hospital.

Complications

Meningitis can cause long-term side-effects, such as deafness, mental handicap and epilepsy, and in some cases may be fatal.

Prevention

Immunisation against Haemophilus Influenza (HIB) has been available since October 1992. It is offered at the same time as immunisation against tetanus, pertussis and diphtheria. There is currently no vaccination against the other forms of meningitis (bacterial or viral).

Infections of the Eye

CONJUNCTIVITIS

Inflammation of the conjunctiva (membrane between the eye and the eyelid) caused by bacteria or virus. (Sometimes conjunctivitis may be the the result of an allergic reaction.)

Characteristics

The child:

- may rub his or her eyes frequently;
- may have a discharge of pus from the corner of the eyes, particularly in the mornings.

The child's:

- eyelids may stick together, particularly after a night's sleep;
- eye may be itchy;
- eye may weep;
- eye will be red.

Specific Care

- The child will need reassurance if the eyelids are stuck together, as he or she may be frightened.
- The carer must wash his or her hands before and after bathing infected eyes. The eyelids should be bathed gently using warm water and cotton wool. Each eye must be wiped from the bridge of the nose outward, and the cotton wool discarded after each wipe.
- The child should be encouraged to keep the eye closed until the pus has been removed.
- The child will need to be seen by a doctor, who may prescribe antibiotic eyedrops if he or she thinks the cause is bacterial. If the cause is allergic or chemical, anti-inflammatory eyedrops may be prescribed.
- If the child is old enough to understand, he or she should be encouraged not to touch the eyes and, if he or she does, to wash the hands afterwards.

Remember, conjunctivitis caused by bacteria or viruses is easily spread, so the child should be kept at home until the condition has improved. Face cloths and towels should never be shared because of the risk of infection.

Infections of the Ear

OTITIS MEDIA

This is an inflammation of the middle ear caused by bacteria or virus.

Young children are more prone to otitis media because of their relatively short Eustachian tube (the tube that connects the throat and the ear). This means that bacteria or viruses in the throat can easily track up into the ear.

Characteristics

The child:

- may recently have developed a cold;
- may appear unwell;
- will usually complain of earache;
- will pull at their ears if unable to indicate the pain verbally;
- may have a raised temperature;
- may vomit;
- may have difficulty with hearing;
- may have pus discharging from the ear (which occurs if the ear drum perforates).

Specific Care

- The child will need to see a doctor, who may prescribe antibiotics and sometimes a decongestant.
- The child will need some paracetamol to relieve the pain.

Complications

Some children suffer from recurrent otitis media may develop glue ear (see below). These children may be referred to an Ear, Nose and Throat (ENT) specialist. The child may need to have grommets inserted.

GLUE EAR

A condition characterised by a build-up of sticky fluid in the middle-ear cavity. This prevents normal vibration of the tympanic membrane and can lead to partial deafness. It occurs most commonly as a complication of otitis media.

Characteristics

The child:

- will usually have a history of repeated ear infections;
- will probably have intermittent hearing loss, which can be very frustrating for both the child and the carer;
- may show a change in behaviour (for example, become very clingy, demanding or disruptive) during these episodes.

The child's:

- speech may be adversely affected (in order to develop a normal speech pattern, children need to hear words clearly – if the sound is frequently muffled, speech may be unclear);
- schoolwork may deteriorate.

Specific Care

- The child will need to see a doctor if glue ear or hearing loss is suspected.
- The doctor may refer the child to a specialist, who will arrange further investigations.
- If severe enough, the specialist may wish to insert grommets into the ear drum to aid the drainage of the fluid and ventilation of the inner ear.
- Insertion of grommets is done under a general anaesthetic, and the child will be admitted to hospital.
- Sometimes the adenoids (lymph tissue found in the nose) are removed at the same time, as they may have been contributing to the cause.
- Advice will need to be taken as to whether the child can get the ears wet after the insertion of grommets (opinions vary).
- If the child has speech difficulties, he or she will be referred to a speech therapist.

Communicating with a Child with a Hearing Loss

- Gain the child's attention before speaking.
- Speak clearly.

- Keep background noise to a minimum.
- Be aware that the child may not hear you.
- Be understanding. The child may be bewildered by intermittent loss of hearing and need your reassurance.

Infections of the Respiratory Tract

THE COMMON COLD

A viral infection of the upper respiratory tract. There are many different viruses that can cause the colds, and the child may be infected several times a year.

Characteristics

The child may:

- have a runny nose;
- have a sore throat;
- have a raised temperature;
- sneeze;
- cough;
- feel generally unwell.

Specific Care

- Make sure that the child has plenty of fluids and rest if unwell.
- Seek medical advice if a baby is having difficulty in feeding or breathing, or you suspect another infection, such as influenza, a chest infection, conjunctivitis or an ear infection.

CROUP

This is a condition characterised by a barking cough. It is usually caused by a virus often associated with the common cold. The virus causes the air passages to swell, and breathing is noisy due to the air passing over the swollen respiratory tubes. Attacks occur more frequently at night. The child may have been well when he or she went to bed.

Characteristics

The child may:

- be hoarse;
- have a barking cough and breathe more rapidly than usual;
- have difficulty breathing and be fighting for breath;
- be distressed;
- wheeze;
- drool saliva.

Remember, the combination of rib recession (when the ribs appear to be sucked in), drooling and difficulty in breathing may indicate that the child is very unwell, and urgent medical assistance should be sought.

Specific Care

- Stay calm. If the carer panics, the child will panic, which will make breathing more difficult.
- Ask someone to ring the doctor (and ambulance, if the child is severely unwell). If there is no one else in the house, pick the child up first and hold him or her while ringing to give reassurance.
- If at any time the child is having serious breathing difficulties, an ambulance must be called. It is advisable to call the doctor as well, as he or she may arrive before the ambulance.
- Take the child to the bathroom, close the windows and steam the room up by filling the bath with hot water. The warm, moist air, together with the closeness of the carer, often results in a great improvement. *Ensure that the child is kept safely away from the hot water.*
- Stay with the child in this atmosphere for approximately twenty minutes.
- If there is a noticeable improvement, take the child back to his or her bed or cot. A parent should sleep in the same room and be prepared to repeat the procedure again if necessary. The doctor will have visited or offered advice by this time.

Infections of the Chest

These are a group of infections, including bronchitis (inflammation of the bronchi due to infection), bronchiolitis (inflammation of the bronchioles due to infection which affects babies and young children) and pneumonia (inflammation of the lung). Although they affect different areas of the lungs, many of the characteristics are similar. They may be caused by bacteria or viruses.

Characteristics

The child:

- may have a chesty cough, initially dry; later, he or she might produce phlegm, which children usually swallow;
- may have a coughing attack, which may result in vomiting;
- often has a raised temperature;
- often has a rapid respiratory rate;
- will look and feel unwell;
- may wheeze;
- may be restless and irritable;
- may have a dry mouth.

Specific Care

- The child will need to see a doctor.
- If the child is having difficulty breathing, he or she will need urgent medical attention and an ambulance will need to be called.
- Encourage the child to take plenty of fluids. If breast fed, the baby should be offered the breast more often.
- Prop the child up if he or she is in bed. Breathing will be easier if the child is held in a sitting position, supported and reassured by the carer.
- Allow plenty of rest and sleep. Running around may start a coughing attack.

TUBERCULOSIS (TB)

A condition in which many areas of the body can be attacked by the bacteria. In the UK, seventy-five per cent of new cases affect the respiratory tract. Other areas that may be affected include the kidneys, meninges (membrane enclosing the brain and spinal cord) or bone. The condition is usually found among immigrant families from areas of the world where TB is more common.

Characteristics

A child with TB lung may:

- be tired;
- lose the appetite;
- lose weight;
- cough;
- have a raised temperature.

Specific Care

The child will be admitted to hospital for initial care. He or she will have various investigations, and once the diagnosis has been confirmed, antibiotic treatment will be started. Antibiotics will be given long term (i.e. up to a year). The child will be reviewed in an outpatient clinic regularly during this time.

Prevention

BCG immunisation is routinely given in some areas of the country at the age of ten to fourteen. Babies born to parents of ethnic background where it is known that the incidence of tuberculosis is high (for example, the Indian subcontinent, parts of Africa and Central and South America) are given a BCG soon after birth.

Infections of the Throat

Tonsillitis

Inflammation of the tonsils, which may be caused by a bacteria or virus.

Characteristics

The child:

- will have a sore throat;
- will have a raised temperature;
- will look and feel unwell;
- will have enlarged tonsils;
- may have unpleasant breath.

Specific Care

- Plenty of rest.
- Fluids should be encouraged – ice lollies are particularly soothing.
- Give pain relief in the form of paediatric paracetamol.
- The child may need to be seen by a doctor, who may prescribe antibiotics. However, the majority of cases are caused by viruses, and the doctor may feel that antibiotics are not appropriate.

Complications

It may be necessary to remove the tonsils (tonsillectomy) if the child suffers repeated attacks of tonsillitis. The child would need to be referred to an Ear, Nose and Throat specialist for advice.

Very rarely it can lead to nephritis (inflammation of the kidney) or rheumatic fever (an infection of the heart).

Infections of the Gastro-Intestinal Tract

ORAL THRUSH

This is a fungal infection of the mouth which affects young babies more frequently than older children.

Characteristics

- White patches inside the mouth, particularly on the gums and tongue, which cannot be wiped off.
- The baby may be reluctant to feed.

Specific Care

The baby will need to be seen by a doctor, who will prescribe treatment.

GASTROENTERITIS

This is a condition where there is inflammation of the stomach and bowel caused by a virus or bacteria.

Characteristics

The child:

- usually has diarrhoea (frequent, loose, offensive bowel motions);
- may vomit;
- often has a raised temperature;
- has a loss of appetite;
- may have abdominal discomfort.

Specific Care

General
- Gastroenteritis can be serious, and the child should be taken to the doctor if the carer is concerned.
- Children with gastroenteritis should stay at home.
- Hygiene must be of a high standard. The infection spreads quickly.
- The child will need reassurance.
- If the child is vomiting, he or she will need lots of reassurance whilst vomiting and afterwards, when they often feel wretched. The carer will need to protect the area around the child to prevent soiling. A bowl should be provided, and the carer will need to stay with the child. After vomiting, the child should be offered a mouthwash if he or she is old enough to co-operate. Clothes should be changed if necessary, and the child should be allowed to rest.
- Small amounts of fluid should be frequently offered; the doctor or health visitor may suggest an electrolyte-replacing mixture to prevent dehydration (see page 104).
- The anal area may become sore – careful washing and the use of a barrier cream will help to prevent this.

For a baby
- Consult the health visitor or doctor. The advice is usually to stop milk feeds. The baby should be offered small amounts of water (preferably mixed with Diarolyte or Rehydrat) at frequent intervals, for example every fifteen to thirty minutes. Diarolyte and Rehydrat can be bought from the chemist without prescription. These are powders that contain glucose and minerals to replace those that are lost through diarrhoea and vomiting. They must be made up as directed.
- Wash the nappy area with care and use a good barrier cream to protect the skin (diarrhoea can chafe the skin, leaving it very sore).
- Nappies should be dealt with carefully, remembering that they

contain infective waste. Hands should be washed with soap and water before and after handling them.

- The baby will need more rest. Keep him or her near you so that you can monitor the situation and be there to help if he or she vomits.
- The baby may be very irritable, this is understandable, so cuddle him or her and keep him or her as comfortable as possible.
- Watch out for signs of dehydration (see below).
- Once the diarrhoea and vomiting has stopped, feeds can be gradually reintroduced. Initially, the feed should be made up at half strength and fed more often than usual, with smaller amounts at each feed; for instance, if the baby usually has 6 oz of feed every four hours, then offer 1½ oz of half-strength feed every hour for a few hours. If this is tolerated, offer 3 oz every two hours and so on, until the half-strength milk is being offered and tolerated at the usual feed times, then gradually reintroduce full-strength milk.
- Breast-fed babies are much less likely to get gastroenteritis. If a breast-fed baby develops gastroenteritis, the carer should discuss the care with the doctor or health visitor.

For older children
- Stop all milk (and milk products) for twenty-four hours.
- Offer Diarolyte or Rehydrat (as above).
- If the child is hungry, offer bland, milk-free foods in small amounts when he or she has stopped vomiting.
- Encourage the child to have plenty of rest.
- Be particularly kind and patient with the child, as he or she may feel embarrassed.
- Gradually reintroduce food and milk; discuss with the health visitor if unsure.
- Watch out for signs of dehydration (see below).

Signs of Dehydration

The child will be thirsty. He or she will pass little or no urine (as a guide, a baby's nappy is usually wet every few hours). Any urine passed will be more concentrated than usual. The tongue and lips will appear to be dry. The skin is less elastic than usual (if you take a small amount of skin on the forearm between the fingers and gently pull the skin up and then let go, it should spring back; if the child is dehydrated, it will take time to go back). The child will be irritable. The eyes will appear to be sunken, as will the fontanelles in a baby. The child lacks energy and may go into a coma.

If these signs are present, the child must be seen by a doctor urgently for assessment.

Complications

Gastroenteritis can, occasionally, lead to loss of body fluids and important minerals (electrolytes) which can, in turn, lead to convulsions, kidney failure, heart irregularities and even death.

APPENDICITIS

This is the inflammation of the appendix; the child may become acutely unwell or the onset may be slower. It is rare in babies and relatively rare in young children.

Characteristics

The child:

- may have pain in the abdomen, initially centrally, but later settling on the lower part of the right side;
- will have a raised temperature;
- will usually have a loss of appetite;
- may vomit;
- may have a change of bowel habit, either diarrhoea or constipation;
- may have bad breath and a dry, coated tongue.

Specific Care

The doctor should be consulted, and the child will probably be admitted to hospital for surgical removal of the appendix.

Complications

If treatment is delayed, the appendix may burst and cause peritonitis (inflammation of the membrane lining the cavity of the abdomen).

Infections of the Urinary Tract

Infections of the urinary tract are common infections seen in children. They occur more in girls than boys.

Characteristics

The child:

- may pass urine more often than usual (the urine may be foul smelling);
- may have pain when passing urine;
- may have lower abdominal pain;
- may have a raised temperature;
- may vomit.

An older child may urgently need to pass urine and may, as a result, be incontinent.

Specific Care

The child will need to be seen by a doctor. A sample of urine will probably be taken – the carer will be shown how to do this. The child may be prescribed antibiotics. The temperature will need to be controlled. The child will be encouraged to drink plenty of fluids. Pain relief, for example paracetamol, may need to be given.

Infections of the Blood

ACQUIRED IMMUNODEFICIENCY SYNDROME (AIDS)

This is an illness caused by infection with the Human Immunodeficiency Virus (HIV). The virus damages the immune defence system, leaving it vulnerable to attack by infective organisms.

Note: if a person has been infected with Human Immunodeficiency Virus but his or her immune system has not been affected, he or she is HIV positive. This person does not have AIDS, although AIDS is likely to develop at some time in the future.

Effects of the Virus

Human Immunodeficiency Virus may enter the body via one of the routes listed on page 107. It then infects the lymphocytes (crucial to the defence against infection). The infected lymphocyte may die, or the virus may lie dormant; if dormant, there may be little or no effect. Sometimes the child may have a mild, flu-like illness and then apparently recover.

The incubation period for the virus is six months to ten years. The virus can be found in blood, semen, breast milk, saliva and urine of infected persons. The following methods of transmission carry a high risk:

- unprotected sex with an infected person;
- via blood (either by intravenous drug users sharing contaminated needles or by a transfusion of infected blood or blood products);
- infected tissue donation;
- an infected mother can pass the disease to the unborn child *in utero* or via infected breast milk.

HIV Facts

A child born to an infected mother will probably have HIV antibodies, since these will have been transferred to the child either just before or during birth. This does not necessarily mean that the child is infected, and it may be up to eighteen months before a definite diagnosis can be made.

Since 1985, the testing of blood in the UK has eliminated transmission of the virus via blood transfusion. However, in some parts of the world, testing is not carried out.

Characteristics

The child with AIDS may:

- be prone to infections, including diarrhoea, mouth infections (particularly thrush) and chest infections;
- have a fever and night sweats due to the infection;
- have enlarged lymph glands;
- lose weight;
- fail to thrive;
- have developmental delay.

Specific Care

There is currently no cure for AIDS, and death may be anticipated eventually. However, treatment can be given to alleviate symptoms, as in any illness; for example, antibiotics for infections and fluid replacement for diarrhoea.

The same principles of care apply to a child with AIDS as with any other sick child. However, at all times particular care must be taken to prevent the spread of the virus to those in contact with the child. When the child is well there should be no reason for him or her to be kept away from school, playschool or other activities.

Protection of Carers and Others

Day-care establishments and hospitals should have a policy for dealing with body fluids which should be followed at all times. The carer may be looking after a child who is HIV positive without any knowledge to that effect.

This policy would include:

- wearing disposable latex gloves when dealing with blood, urine and vomit;
- using one per cent hypochlorite solution to cover any blood spillages. The area should then be wiped over with a gloved hand using disposable cloths, which should then be discarded into a bag and sent for incineration. The area should then be washed with hot, soapy water;
- washing the hands after dealing with spillages (even if gloves have been used);
- avoiding sharp instruments that could result in injury;
- covering cuts or grazes with a waterproof plaster.

If a carer punctures his or her skin, and there is a possibility that any body fluid has been in contact with the punctured area, the carer must thoroughly wash the area with soapy water and encourage the puncture to bleed. He or she must then seek urgent medical advice. An accident form must also be completed.

HEPATITIS

Inflammation of the liver, caused in most cases by one of two viruses.

Type A virus causes hepatitis A (infective hepatitis) which has an incubation period of ten to forty days.

108

Type B virus causes hepatitis B (serum hepatitis) which has an incubation period of sixty to 160 days.

Characteristics

The child may:

- feel tired;
- feel generally unwell;
- lose his or her appetite;
- have a raised temperature;
- be jaundiced;
- have dark urine and pale stools.

Hepatitis B can be transmitted in similar ways to HIV. The policy on protection of carers as described for HIV (see page 108) applies equally to hepatitis B.

Specific Care

- The child will need to be seen by the doctor.
- The child should be cared for at home (or in hospital, if the doctor advises).
- Rest is very important.
- Encourage the child to drink plenty of fluids.
- Scrupulous hygiene is vitally important, as this is an extremely infectious disease. Ideally, the child should be cared for in his or her own room and he or she must use only personal towels, which should be kept separate from others. If there is more than one toilet in the house, this should be allocated for the child's personal use; if not, extremely thorough hygienic practices will need to be used.

Complications

The child may feel unwell for many months after the infection; once free of infection, he or she may feel well one day and poorly the next. He or she may therefore have to return to school/playgroup on a part-time basis.

Hepatitis B can cause death through liver failure.

A number of people who have had hepatitis B remain carriers. A carrier is someone who does not suffer from the infection, but who is capable of passing the infection to others.

Vaccination against hepatitis B is available for people who are particularly at risk, for instance health workers.

Infections of the Skin

These can be caused by:

- bacteria, such as impetigo;
- viruses, such as warts and verrucas;
- fungi, such as ringworm;
- insects, such as scabies;
- worms, such as toxocara.

IMPETIGO

Impetigo is an infection of the skin caused by bacteria that most commonly affects the face (although it can affect other parts of the body). It is easily spread by contact with infected flannels and towels.

Characteristics

The child may initially have small blisters which break down, leaving weeping areas which crust over.

Specific Care

- It is highly infectious, and the child should therefore be cared for at home.
- Separate face cloths and towels should be used for each member of the family (as always).
- The carer should wash his or her hands after touching the face.
- The child should be encouraged to leave the crusts alone.
- The child will need to see a doctor, who will usually prescribe antibiotics. He or she will also advise when the child can start mixing with other children again.

Complications

These are uncommon, but if the condition is untreated, generalised infection may result.

WARTS

Warts appears as raised lumps on the surface of the skin. They can occur all over the body and can be spread by direct contact with an infected person.

Warts will eventually disappear, but sometimes treatment is desirable because of pain or unsightliness. Various treatments are available over the counter at the chemists, usually in the form of a weak acid. However, these must be used with care, as they may cause the surrounding skin to be burned. If unsuccessful, the wart may be treated by freezing with liquid nitrogen – so-called cryosurgery – but again, some discomfort is almost inevitable, so many doctors may advise a 'wait-and-see' approach.

A verruca is simply a wart that, by virtue of its position on the sole of the foot, has been pushed inwards. Treatment is the same as for warts. It is sometimes recommended that the child wears a rubber sock to prevent the spread of the infection when swimming.

ATHLETE'S FOOT OR RINGWORM

Athlete's foot is a fungal infection that particularly affects the areas between the toes, a habitat in which the fungus thrives. It is infectious and can be transmitted in shower areas and swimming pools. The child will complain of itchy feet, particularly between the toes, where the skin will be found to be pink and flaky. The intense itching – and hence scratching – may lead to bleeding.

The doctor will prescribe treatment, usually in the form of a powder or a cream. If the carer is worried that the condition has not cleared up as expected or that the child's nails have become infected, a doctor should be consulted again.

The carer should carefully wash and dry between the child's toes each day. Ideally, socks should be of cotton material, and shoes made of natural material should be worn. The child should keep the feet covered when walking around the house. Each member of the family should have separate towels.

Ringworm is a fungal infection of the skin, which appears as a red ring. It can also affect the scalp, where it may cause bald patches. The infection can be passed from animals to people, but more usually it passes from person to person. The child will need to be seen by the doctor, who will prescribe treatment.

111

Prevention of spread is effected by washing hands thoroughly after touching the area and using separate towels and flannels. If the infection came from an animal, it should be taken to a vet for treatment.

HEAD LICE

The head louse is an insect which lives on the scalp; although it can be seen by the naked eye, it has a tendency to appear the same colour as the hair, making it difficult to find. The adult lays eggs on the shaft of the hair close to the root. These eggs are called nits; they are small, oval-shaped structures, which at first glance look like dandruff. Unlike dandruff, though, they are very firmly attached to the hair.

Once the egg has hatched, the insect bites the scalp and causes intense itching.

The lice can transfer from one head to another very easily by direct contact and they are not choosy about the type of hair they infest. If a child has head lice, treatment should be carried out as soon as possible. The carer should note that treatments change frequently because head lice are masters at developing resistance to treatments, and the health visitor, doctor or pharmacist should therefore be consulted before treating.

Once treated, the louse can no longer cause harm, and the child can return to his or her usual routine. It is important that members of the same family, or those in close contact with the child, should be inspected and treated as necessary.

Prevention of infestation is not easy because of the close proximity in which young children play and work, which allows easy transmission.

However children should be encouraged to brush their hair thoroughly each day, as this will break the legs of the lice, making it impossible for them to lay their eggs near the base of the hair.

SCABIES

Scabies is a condition caused by the skin becoming infested by an insect. This insect burrows into the skin, where it lays its eggs and causes intense itching. A red rash appears around the infected areas. Scabies is transmitted by direct contact.

Scabies is most commonly found between the fingers, but may also be found in the palms, wrists, armpits, soles of the feet and genital area.

The child should be seen by a doctor, who will prescribe treatment. (Treatments can be bought over the counter at the chemists, but they may not be suitable for children.) It is usually recommended that the whole family is treated at the same time because of the likelihood of spread to close contacts.

THREADWORMS

Threadworms are small, white worms that can infest the bowel. Infection occurs when the eggs are ingested. These are usually picked up on hands and will be ingested if the child puts the hands in the mouth. The eggs are very small and can be passed from one person to another via bed linen, towels, clothing or unwashed vegetables and soil.

Threadworms are contagious and easily pass from one person to another. They cause itching around the anus, particularly at night. The child will scratch, eggs will be caught under the nails and the cycle may repeat itself.

Treatment will be prescribed by the doctor. The whole family should be treated at the same time.

Prevention is through meticulous food and personal hygiene, which includes the use of separate towels, scrubbing the nails after a bowel movement and keeping the child's nails short.

TOXOCARIASIS

Toxocariasis is a condition that can occur if the eggs of the toxocara worm are ingested.

The toxicara worm lives in the gut of dogs and cats, and the eggs of the worm are excreted in their faeces. If young children play in an area where dogs and cats have fouled the soil, they may come into contact with the faeces. Young children are particularly at risk because they often put their hands in their mouths and thereby ingest the eggs.

After ingestion, the eggs hatch in the gut and then pass through the intestinal wall. They make their way to the liver and other organs in the body.

This may cause the child to become unwell, with a raised temperature, rash and they feel poorly. As the larvae migrate, they can cause bleeding and infection. In severe infections, inflammation of the optic nerve may occur, and blindness may result.

If there is a suspicion that the child has been in contact with excreta in this way, a doctor should be consulted for advice and tests if appropriate.

Prevention is through public education. All dog and cat owners should regularly worm their animals. Dogs should be prevented from entering children's playgrounds by dog-proof fencing.

STUDENT ACTIVITIES

Common Infectious Diseases
I   Write a fact sheet for parents entitled 'Prevention of the spread of infection'.

Protection of Carers and Others
I   You may not yet have seen a written policy for spillages in the workplace. Working in a group, imagine you are working in a day nursery. Write a policy for the workplace. Consider, for instance, where you will keep the gloves; if they are kept in a central location, they may not be accessible when needed. Where will you store your one per cent hypochlorite solution? How will you ensure that the discarded material is incinerated? Where will it go whilst waiting for incineration?

Toxocariasis
I   You have recently been appointed as a nanny. The family has three children under the age of five. They own three cats. You have been asked for advice on worming these cats. Find out from the local veterinary surgery the current recommendations.

Head Lice
I   You are working in a day nursery. Over the last few weeks, many children have been affected by head lice. You have informed the parents of the affected children and asked them to treat their children. However, you feel that it would be worthwhile to run a teaching session for all parents. You have decided to keep the session short – just fifteen minutes. Write to the Health Education Unit in your area and ask for a copy of any leaflets on the subject; they may also have some teaching materials you could review. The health visitor may have some further information and be pleased to discuss the project with you.

Once you have completed your research, prepare your session. Consider the handouts you might use, any visual aids, such as an overhead projector, posters or perhaps a videotape. Consider when you might run this session to enable as many parents or carers to attend as possible. Consider also the care of the children in the day nursery whilst this session is being run; make sure that enough staff are available to care for the children.

10

ACCIDENTAL INJURIES

—

'An accident is an unpremeditated event resulting in recognisable damage.'
World Health Organisation

An accident is something that happens unexpectedly, so the carer must ensure he or she has done everything possible to prevent it. Accidents are the most common cause of death in children aged between one and fourteen. In 1989, more than 800 children were killed in accidents in the United Kingdom. Accidents are also responsible for many disabilities.

Why Do They Happen?

Children are naturally curious about their environment and are prone to accidents because of their inexperience and their ever-increasing mobility and manipulative skills.

It is the carer's responsibility to protect the child from danger. In order to do this, he or she must have a thorough understanding of normal growth and development. He or she must be aware of the child's normal milestones and how any particular child compares to the norm. He or she will then always be ready for the next stage and will therefore, as far as possible, provide the necessary protection.

The Role of the Child Carer in the Prevention of Accidents

The carer must:

- try to see the world through the eyes of a child and therefore anticipate potential accidents;

115

FIRE RESISTANT FURNITURE

SAFETY MARK (BRITISH STANDARDS INSTITUTION – FOUND ON GAS COOKERS AND OTHER GAS APPLIANCES)

BEAB MARK (FOUND ON ELECTRICAL GOODS)

KITEMARK (BRITISH STANDARDS INSTITUTION)

LION MARK (FOUND ONLY ON BRITISH-MADE TOYS; THEY WILL HAVE A CE MARK AS WELL)

CE MARK (FOUND ON TOYS WHOSE MANUFACTURER CLAIMS THEY MEET EUROPEAN AND BRITISH TOY SAFETY STANDARDS)

TOXIC SUBSTANCE

CORROSIVE SUBSTANCE

HARMFUL OR IRRITANT SUBSTANCES

HIGHLY FLAMMABLE SUBSTANCES

Figure 22   Safety symbols

- be aware of safety aspects in the child's environment at all times (this may involve some initial training by the parent or the person in charge, followed by regular updating);
- take opportunities to educate those in their care and other carers about safety;
- be observant and spot the safety problems before the child experiences them;
- check equipment regularly – any equipment that has been damaged should be discarded if unrepairable and new equipment should be checked for one of the symbols shown in figure 22;
- plan the indoor/outdoor play layout with safety in mind;
- store equipment safely;
- ensure the child's clothes are safe;
- see him or herself as a role model. All the carer's actions should have safety in mind, so if cycling, he or she should wear a helmet and reflective clothing; if travelling in a car, he or she should ensure that both driver and passengers are appropriately restrained and always drive within speed limits; in the workplace, the carer should wear gloves when dealing with spillages. There should always be an Accident and Health and Safety book on the premises.

Causes of Accidents

There are many causes of accidents, both fatal and otherwise. The most common are shown below in figure 23.

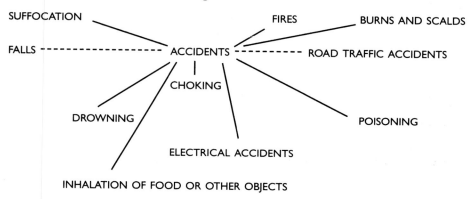

Figure 23   *Common causes of accidents*

Accidents in the Home

The majority of accidents to children under the age of three occur in the home. There are approximately 200 deaths from accidents in the home each year, see figure 24 below.

FATAL ACCIDENTS IN THE HOME (OFFICE OF POPULATION CENSUSES AND SURVEYS, 1989)

AGE	0–4	5–14	ALL CHILDREN	%
TYPE OF ACCIDENT				
FIRES	71	28	99	45
CHOKING	43	7	50	23
DROWNING	20	3	23	10
FALLS	12	7	19	9
POISONING	5	4	9	4
HOT SUBSTANCES	5	2	7	3
ELECTRICAL	2	0	2	1
OTHER	11	1	12	5

Note: carers would be advised to attend a first-aid course, which would enable them to deal with the initial care of a child who has been involved in any of these accidents.

STUDENT ACTIVITIES

Fires and burns
1   On the first day of work experience or in a new job, find out the following:

   • the position of fire-fighting equipment;
   • the position of the telephone;
   • the position of the first-aid box and its contents;
   • the position of the fire exits.

(Always be aware of the importance of keeping the class register up to date so that children can be accounted for if evacuation is necessary.)

Choking and inhalation of food
1   Each year there are a number of children who choke as a result of eating nuts. Find out at what stage nuts can safely be introduced into the child's diet and the reasons for the advice.

Drowning

I   Draw a map of your workplace and surrounding area and mark the high-risk areas for drowning. What measures will you take to prevent a child from drowning?

Falls and cuts

I   Find out the workplace policy for the treatment of cuts and read pages 106–108 to ensure you have a knowledge of prevention of the transmission of HIV.

Poisoning

I   List the possible substances in the workplace and the outside play area that are potentially poisonous. How will you ensure they are not accessible to children?

Accidents on the road

I   Road traffic accidents account for many accidental deaths. The children may be car passengers, cyclists or pedestrians. When crossing the road, squat down and see and hear what the situation looks like from a child's point of view.

Children in cars

I   Find out about the recommended car restraints for children. Make sure that you know how to place the child safely in the restraint.

Suffocation

I   Find out the most common causes of suffocation in children. What is your role in the prevention of these accidents?

The role of the carer

I   Design a leaflet that can be used by all child carers. The leaflet will be divided up as follows:

- prevention of head injuries in the home: 0–6 months
                                                                    6–18 months
                                                                    18 months to 5 years
                                                                    5 years to 8 years
- prevention of head injuries in the garden: 0–6 months
                                                                    7–18 months
                                                                    18 months to 5 years
                                                                    5 years to 8 years
- prevention of head injuries elsewhere, on the road, in the supermarket, in cars and on bicycles.

If possible, work in a group for the production of this leaflet.

Road safety

1   Plan a ten-minute talk to be given in assembly to children aged between five and eight on road safety.

11

ENVIRONMENTAL FACTORS AFFECTING HEALTH

—

There are two types of environment in relation to health – external (outside the body) and internal (within).

The External Environment

ALLERGIES AND THE ALLERGIC REACTION

An allergic reaction occurs when a foreign substance, usually a protein, causes the immune system to over-react in a harmful way. This foreign protein is called an allergen (or an antigen) and it stimulates excessive production of certain types of antibodies.

* An allergic response does not usually occur on the first occasion the body is exposed to the allergen, but may occur after subsequent exposure.
* The foreign substance may be inhaled, ingested or enter via the skin.
* Allergies tend to run in families.

Common allergies include asthma and eczema.

Asthma

Asthma is a condition in which there is intermittent narrowing of the respiratory tubes due to an allergic response. There is often a family history of asthma, eczema or hay fever.

The allergen irritates cells of the respiratory tract to produce a chemical (histamine), causing muscle constriction (bronchospasm), swelling and increased mucus secretion. The air passages are therefore considerably narrowed.

As the airways become increasingly narrowed, breathing becomes more difficult. The characteristic wheeze may also be heard as the child

121

breathes out and is sometimes heard when the child breathes in. At least one in ten children are affected in Britain.

Causes (sometimes called trigger factors)
Asthma is often associated with an allergic response and can be triggered by:

- exposure to an inhaled antigen, such as pollen, the house dust mite (which lives on shed human skin) or animal fur;
- infections, such as the common cold;
- exercise;
- emotion, excitement or stress;
- (some children are sensitive to cigarette smoke or to fumes from various substances, such as car exhaust);
- cold air;
- food.

Recent research indicates that air pollution is also likely to be a cause.

Effects on the child
The onset of an attack may be gradual or abrupt. In general, if the attack is in response to an infection, onset is gradual. If it is in response to an antigen, it will have an acute onset. The child will have a cough, which initially is dry, irritating and unproductive and is characteristically worse at night. Later, the child may cough up and swallow small amounts of thick sticky mucus. The child may become breathless, and the wheeze can be heard as the child breathes out through these narrowed airways. He or she is often very frightened at this stage and may sweat and appear pale. The older child may sit up, thus trying to increase the area for air entry.

If the carer looks at the chest at this stage, he or she may observe that the child is breathing more rapidly than usual and may have some rib recession. The child may have difficulty speaking. A child who has rapid respiration, difficulty speaking and rib recession needs to be seen urgently by a doctor.

Care of the child
If this is the first episode or if the carer is worried about the child at any stage in the course of the attack, medical help should be requested.

- Stay calm – the child is likely to be anxious.
- Stay with the child, reassure him or her and avoid fussing.

- Try not to ask too many questions which need responses. The child may be using all available energy for breathing.
- Children often find the sitting position the most comfortable, supported with pillows as necessary. A younger child will probably find it more comforting to sit on the carer's lap.

A child who is known to have asthma will usually have treatment with him or her, which should be given as directed by the parents. If there is little or no response to the treatment, medical advice should be requested. In some cases it may be necessary to telephone for an ambulance. If the child is away from his or her parents, they should be telephoned and asked to return, because ill children are usually best reassured by their parents. Warm fluids may soothe the throat and help the child feel a little better. Try to distract the child, for example by reading a story. This may decrease the anxiety.

Treatment
Bronchodilator drugs (sometimes called 'relievers') work on the muscles in the airways to open up or dilate them and thus help in the reversal process. Commonly prescribed bronchodilators include Ventolin (Salbutamol) and Bricanyl (Terbutaline). They can be given via an inhaler or orally. Inhalation is the preferred method, as this has the advantage of working directly on the respiratory tract and therefore results in fewer side-effects. Recently, 'spacer devices' have been used for children. These have the advantage of enabling the child to inhale the medication without needing the careful co-ordination required by other inhalers. If the bronchodilator is not effective, medical assistance should be requested. The doctor may administer the bronchodilator through a nebuliser. This is a machine that delivers the dose up in a fine mist, which is delivered via a mask.

Steroids may be given in an acute attack. They have powerful anti-inflammatory properties and will complement the bronchodilators. If the child fails to respond to the treatment, he or she may need to be admitted to hospital. The child will already be frightened and should be kept as calm as possible. Ideally, the parent(s) or carer should stay with him or her.

Preventative treatment
This will be considered if the child has frequent or severe episodes of wheezing.

The child may be prescribed:

- Intal (sodium chromoglycate) given via an inhaler; this must be given regularly as directed;
- inhaled steroids, for example Becotide;
- the doctor may suggest that the child takes a dose of the bronchodilator before exercise, particularly if this is known to cause wheezing.

The child and carer are often asked to measure and record the child's peak flow reading (which indirectly measures the airway narrowing). Readings taken while the child is well will form a basis for the normal reading for that child. During an asthmatic attack, the readings will drop and give the doctor an objective measurement of the severity of the attack. Sometimes the doctor devises an action or care plan for the child. This is organised so that the carer knows what action to take if the peak flow drops and at what stage medical help should be sought.

Eczema

Eczema is characterised by dry, itchy skin – red, rough areas may be seen. It affects up to one in ten children. There are two main types of eczema: atopic eczema and seborrhoeic eczema.

Atopic eczema

Atopic eczema is the most common type seen in children. There is often a family history of eczema and/or hay fever and asthma.

It is uncommon for a child to develop atopic eczema before the age of three months. Generally, forty per cent of children have grown out of it by the age of two years and ninety per cent by teenage years.

Effects of the child

The condition is characterised by periods of remissions and relapses. The skin is dry and scaly. When there is a relapse of the condition, there is intense itching, which is worse at night and may cause sleep disturbance. This leads to scratching. The skin becomes red and inflamed. Fluid filled vesicles may appear on the skin and these tear and weep when scratched. This leads to loss of fluid and the child feels very thirsty. The fluid dries on the skin and forms a crusty exudate. The torn skin can be an entry for infection, which is a frequent complication of eczema. Later, there may be some loss of pigmentation of the skin and it may go on to have a leathery appearance.

Care of the child and treatment

Treatment is aimed at decreasing the itching and combating the dryness of the skin; this is usually achieved by the use of moisturising and steroid creams. Moisturising cream should be applied to the body at least twice a day. Several moisturisers may be used; the doctor and carer may have to try several before the best one for the individual is found.

- Moisturising creams should be used regularly during the day, for instance aqueous cream or E45 cream.
- Emollients are oily preparations that are soothing to the skin and should be added to the bath water. They are usually prescribed by the doctor. Some need to be dissolved in boiling water before being added to the bath water. Soap should be avoided because it tends to dry the skin and, if perfumed, may itself be an allergen. Soap substitutes include aqueous cream, which is available over the counter at the chemist or on prescription. The bath water should be tepid – never hot, as the heat is an irritant. Sometimes it is advised not to bath the child every day because of the general drying nature of bath water.
- Steroid creams or ointments need to be prescribed by the doctor. (Steroid creams or ointments are anti-inflammatory and they decrease the allergic reaction.) The weakest cream that is effective should be used and it should be used sparingly. The carer must use them as instructed and must wash his or her hands after use, as the cream or ointment may be absorbed and cause unwanted effects in the carer. Sometimes the carer is advised to wear protective gloves when applying these creams.
- Antihistamines may be prescribed because of their anti-itch properties and because they are not addictive. They are particularly useful at night because of their sedative properties, which allow the child to get some sleep.
- Tar preparations are sometimes used for stubborn cases.

General management that helps

- Pure cotton clothing is cool and absorbent.
- Avoid overheating the room – children with eczema feel more comfortable and itch less if they are cared for in cool temperatures. They should avoid direct sunlight and any direct heat.
- Clothes should be washed in non-biological washing powders, and fabric softeners should be avoided.

125

- Usually no dietary restrictions are necessary, but sometimes a doctor may feel that it is worthwhile trying a special diet, for example the elimination of milk and milk-based products. This must, however, be tried with the supervision of a dietician.

Sometimes children with skin complaints may be teased by their peers. The carer must be aware of this possibility and deal with any problems.

Prevention
There is no known prevention for eczema, but it is recognised that breast feeding a baby up to four to six months is beneficial in the avoidance of allergy.

Complications
Infections of the skin can occur because of the scratching. The child may require antibiotics from the doctor, either as ointments, creams or orally. Infections of the skin should be prevented as far as possible by discouraging scratching and ensuring the finger nails are kept clean and short. If the child scratches at night, it may be a good idea to put cotton mitts on the hands at bedtime. It is also a good idea to use cotton pyjamas that fasten together where the top and the bottom meet.

The condition can put a strain on the whole family if the affected child has disturbed nights. This can cause stress and poor performance at work or at school.

The Internal Environment

The internal environment is, in part, controlled by the endocrine glands which secrete hormones directly into the blood stream. Hormones are chemicals released in one part of the body that have an effect in another part. These endocrine glands can potentially go out of control and either not secrete enough hormone or release too much.

Hormones are secreted from the pituitary gland, the thyroid gland, the parathyroid glands, the adrenal glands and the ovaries or testes and the Islets of Langerhans in the pancreas.

DIABETES

Diabetes is a condition in which there is insufficient insulin produced by the pancreas, resulting in the blood sugar level being higher than normal. There are two types of diabetes. The first is called insulin-dependent diabetes. In this type, the patient requires injections of insulin – this is the type that affects children.

The second type is called non-insulin-dependent diabetes and is controlled by medication and diet, or diet alone. This is more common than the former type, but not often seen in children.

Cause

The cause of diabetes is unknown; however, it does occur more often than might be expected in families (that is, it is familial). It is thought that a viral infection at an earlier stage in life may have acted as a trigger. In the UK, approximately one child in 1000 develops insulin-dependent diabetes.

The Effect on the Child

Sugar needs to be absorbed from the blood in order to be used by the cells. The signs and symptoms of diabetes arise because the sugar in the blood cannot be utilised by the body.

Raised levels of blood sugar lead to:

- sugar in the urine (glycosuria). This occurs because the kidney tubules cannot reabsorb the large quantities of sugar from the urine. This in turn leads to:
- large amounts of urine being passed (polyuria) causing:
- thirst (polydipsia) to compensate for the polyuria.

To try to compensate for the lack of energy available from sugar, the body breaks down fat and protein. The breakdown of fat and protein leads to weight loss, increased appetite and tiredness. When fats are broken down and used, ketones are released, and these may leave a characteristic smell like pear drops on the child's breath.

Sometimes the condition develops quickly, and the child may become dehydrated due to the polyuria. The child may also lose consciousness.

If diabetes is suspected, a blood test will confirm a raised blood sugar level. Urine testing will usually confirm sugar in the urine and ketones may be present.

127

Care of the Child

The child will be admitted to hospital for the initial treatment and stabilisation of the condition. The care is based on the balance of insulin, diet and exercise.

Insulin

Whilst in hospital, the child will be assessed to determine the amount of insulin he or she will need. The hormone insulin is injected – it cannot be given orally, because it would be digested before it had an effect. Hospital staff teach the parents (and child, if old enough) to measure and inject insulin and to test the blood sugar level. The parents will learn to measure the correct amount of insulin in the syringe (the dosage will be prescribed by the doctor). Insulin is prescribed in units, so a special insulin syringe, gun or pen is used.

They also need to know the importance of rotating the injection sites to prevent thickening of tissues. The areas that are used as injection sites include the arms, thighs, hips and abdomen (see figure 25).

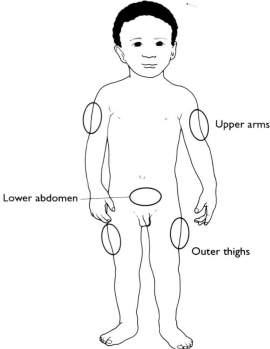

Figure 25   Injection sites for insulin

They also need to learn how to clean and store the insulin syringe, and the importance of storage of the insulin itself. They will be taught to test the blood sugar level at regular intervals. The blood sugar levels should be kept as normal as possible so that the child can avoid complications. They will be taught how to test the urine for sugar and recognise symptoms of high blood sugar level attacks (hyperglycaemia) and low blood sugar level attacks (hypoglycaemic) (see below).

Diet
A dietician will advise the parents on the importance of providing a well-balanced diet. He or she will usually suggest that the child is given three meals and three snacks a day. Specific advice is given to families to meet the individual needs.

Exercise
Exercise should not be restricted. However, it may be necessary to take in more food before strenuous exercise. Medical advice should be followed.

Hypoglycaemia (too little blood sugar)

The causes of hypoglycaemia are:

- too little food;
- too much insulin without adequate food intake;
- too much exercise without food support.

Characteristics
The onset is rapid. The child may become increasingly irritable and lack concentration. He or she may be sweaty and/or dizzy, complain of a headache, vomit and may lapse into unconsciousness.

Once these features have been recognised, steps should be taken quickly to reverse the situation. All diabetics are encouraged to carry a sugary snack or drink with them, which should be taken if the child is conscious.

If the child has lost consciousness, a doctor and an ambulance should be called, and the situation treated as an emergency. The child's parents should be informed of all hypoglycaemia attacks.

Prolonged hypoglycaemia can cause brain damage, as the brain depends on glucose for normal functioning.

Hyperglycaemia (too much blood sugar)

The causes of hyperglycaemia are:

- too little insulin;
- illness, such as infections.

Characteristics

Hyperglycaemia attacks come on slowly. A child will have similar symptoms as described under *The Effect on the Child* see page 127, i.e. the child will feel thirsty, will pass large amounts of urine, will feel sleepy and the breath will smell of pear drops. He or she will feel hot and dry and may feel sick. The child may become unconscious if these symptoms are not recognised. The child must see a doctor urgently. If the child is not with his or her parents, they should be informed.

Complications

Complications other than hyperglycaemia or hypoglycaemia tend to occur later in life. They can be prevented to a large extent by careful management of the condition. The complications are mainly associated with the narrowing of arteries by fatty deposits, which can have an effect on the heart, kidneys, nerves and eyes.

Conclusion

The carer of a diabetic child should:

- be observant for signs of increased thirst, hunger and frequency of passing urine;
- seek expert help if the child is unwell because the diabetes may become out of control;
- inform the parents if any infection is noted;
- inform parents of any problem with eyesight, as diabetics are more prone to sight problems than non-diabetics;
- be aware that the sleeping child may be unconscious, particularly if he or she is sleeping at an unusual time of the day and is sweating, or hot and dry;
- *if the job description demands*, be able to test urine and/or blood for sugar content;
- build high standards of hygiene into daily care and be more disciplined regarding timing and quantity of meals;
- follow the recommended dietary intake;
- monitor the amount of exercise taken.

GROWTH DEFICIENCY

The pituitary gland controls many of the other endocrine glands. It also secretes growth hormone which, if there are deficient amounts, will lead to growth stunting.

There are many causes of growth deficiency, and the child will be referred for assessment and treated with injections of growth hormone if necessary.

Hypothyroidism

The thyroid gland secretes thyroxine. Low levels of thyroxine cause hypothyroidism. The condition is routinely screened for, six days after birth when the Guthrie test is taken. Treatment prevents stunting of mental and physical growth.

STUDENT ACTIVITIES

Diabetes

Design a leaflet of no more than six sides of A4 paper entitled 'I have diabetes'. It should be aimed at children under seven years old and contain the following information: a definition of diabetes; a description of how the child may have felt before being diagnosed; the treatment and tests; recognition of hypoglycaemia and hyperglycaemia.

The student might like to think of a well-known fairy story and base the information on it. The pictures and written work must take into account the child's age and expected stage of development.

Allergies and allergic reactions

1 Prepare an information card for primary school teachers which includes the following information:

- how to deal with an asthmatic attack;
- the action of preventers and relievers;
- the correct way inhalers should be used.

2 You are working as a nursery nurse alongside a health visitor. A child aged two-and-a-half has severe eczema. Unfortunately, he has got into the habit of scratching when he is not occupied. The health visitor has asked you to plan activities for the child that will distract him from scratching, so that

some of the time he is playing with another adult and some of the time he is playing alone supervised by an adult.

Write up your plan in the form of a report that you will give to the health visitor.

12

CONGENITAL FACTORS AFFECTING HEALTH

A congenital abnormality is present at birth. Congenital abnormalities may occur as a result of inherited factors, as well as a number of other factors which are less clear cut. Infection, medication, cigarette smoking and alcohol intake during pregnancy are examples of known causes of congenital abnormality.

Congenital abnormalities may be identified prenatally at birth or in the first year of life, when they may be picked up at the child surveillance clinics.

Genetic Inheritance

In the nucleus of each cell, there are forty-six chromosomes arranged in twenty-three pairs. Half of the chromosomes have come from the mother and half from the father.

Each chromosome has thousands of genes on it, and these carry the information for individual characteristics or development. A gene that controls a specific feature is found in the same place on the same chromosome in each individual.

The individual has two genes for each characteristic; these will usually complement each other, but sometimes one is stronger than the other and is referred to as the dominant gene, the weaker one being referred to as the recessive gene. A relatively straightforward example of dominant and recessive genes is that of eye colour. Brown eye colour is usually a dominant gene and blue eye colour a recessive gene. If both parents have brown eyes, and have inherited two genes for brown eyes from their parents, then all children of these parents will have brown eyes. This is represented in figure 26.

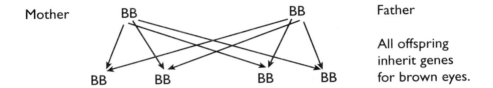

Figure 26   Inheritance (1)   Brown eye colour where both parents have brown eyes and have inherited dominant genes.

If both parents have brown eyes and each inherited one dominant brown gene and one recessive blue gene from their parents, of four possible offspring, there is a one in four chance that a child will have brown eyes, having inherited dominant genes from both parents, a one in four chance that a child will have blue eyes, having inherited recessive genes from both parents, and a one in two chance that two children will have brown eyes having inherited one dominant gene and one recessive gene (see figure 27).

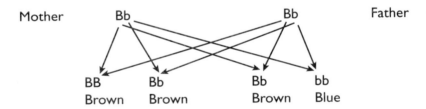

Figure 27   Inheritance (2)   Brown/blue eye colour where both parents have brown eyes and have inherited one dominant brown-eye gene and one recessive blue-eye gene. One child has brown eyes (two dominant genes), two children have brown eyes (one dominant, one recessive gene), one child has blue eyes (two recessive genes).

These examples are relatively straightforward; however, they provide a good example of inheritance, which is usually more complex than eye colouring. Of the twenty-three pairs of chromosomes, twenty-two pairs are autosomes (i.e. they have the same functions and have a similar appearance). The twenty-third pair are the sex chromosomes. They are dissimilar and are referred to as the X chromosome and the Y chromosome. A female will have two X chromosomes, and a male will have an X and a Y chromosome.

Some characteristics are inherited through sex-linked inheritance. The X chromosome carries more genes than the Y chromosome, which is smaller. Some diseases, such as haemophilia, can be inherited by a male if the mother is a carrier (i.e. if the mother has inherited the recessive gene for haemophilia from one parent). If he inherits the X chromosome carrying the affected gene, there is no matching gene on the Y chromosome, and the boy will therefore have the disease.

Genetic Counselling

A couple may be referred to a genetic counsellor:

- if they have an inherited disease;
- if there is a member of the family with an inherited disease;
- if there is a possibility of one of the couple being a carrier.

The genetic counsellor will discuss risks of congenital abnormalities that are inherited or familial (run in families).

MUTATIONS

Mutations can occur. This is when an abnormality is not present in either of the parents, yet the child displays it. Fortunately this is uncommon.

Extra Chromosomes

Sometimes a chromosome does not divide properly, and both chromosomes of a pair may end up in the ova or the sperm. Once fertilised, there will be three chromosomes where there should be a pair. This is called trisomy, and an example of this chromosomal defect is Down's syndrome, which is the result of trisomy 21.

ABNORMALITIES OF DOMINANT GENES

Fortunately, this method of inheritance is not very common. An example is Huntington's chorea, features of this condition are not seen in childhood.

ABNORMALITIES OF RECESSIVE GENES

Cystic Fibrosis

This is the most common genetic disease, affecting one in 2000 births. Approximately one person in twenty carries the abnormal gene.

This condition affects the lungs and the pancreas particularly. The secretions produced are thicker and stickier than usual. In the lungs, this results in small air passages becoming blocked and eventually infected. The child therefore suffers from repeated chest infections.

The child will need physiotherapy at regular intervals during the day. The parents or carer are usually taught to do this. The aim is to loosen the secretions so that they may be coughed up. Antibiotics are prescribed whenever the lungs are infected. Sometimes the repeated chest infections can cause a resistance to blood flow in the lungs, which in turn affects the heart which has to work harder. This can lead to heart failure, and for these children a heart and lung transplant is needed.

In the pancreas, the secretions prevent the digestive enzymes from working efficiently on food to break it down for absorption. This results in food not being absorbed and eventually to a lack of weight gain and possibly failure to thrive. Fat absorption is a particular problem; fat is needed for energy and for the absorption of some vitamins. Unabsorbed fat leaves the gut in its relatively undigested state, making the stools fatty and offensive.

Pancreatic enzymes must be given so that the food can be absorbed and these are given orally with each meal. The child also needs regular vitamin supplements.

Phenylketonuria

Approximately one in 14,000 babies is affected. This is a disorder in which the baby is unable to metabolise the amino acid (a basic unit of protein) phenylalanine. Failure to do so results in a build-up in the bloodstream. Its accumulation prevents normal development of the brain and central nervous system, causing mental handicap. A Guthrie test (a heel prick that allows a small amount of blood to be collected) is routinely done on all babies at about six days old. Babies who are found to have the disorder need to have a dietary restriction of phenylalanine from two weeks of life if it is to be effective in the prevention of mental handicap.

136

Sickle Cell Disease

A disorder mainly affecting people of Afro-Caribbean origin (approximately one in 200), although it can be found in people from the Mediterranean, Asia and Middle East. The haemoglobin in the red blood cell forms a sickle shape when it gives up oxygen under certain conditions, which can result in the cells clumping together as they pass through the blood vessels. (Usually red blood cells remain round when they release oxygen, and this allows them to flow freely through the blood vessels.) The blockage of blood (sickle cell crisis) can cause damage, for example to bone. A crisis (when acute symptoms occur) may be brought on by strenuous exercise, infection, dehydration, pregnancy or an anaesthetic and may cause the child to have a fit or become unconscious.

It is uncommon for the child to have any problems before the age of six months.

In a crisis the child may have the following signs or symptoms.

Pain
This is caused by the cells clumping in the blood vessels and blocking them. This pain may be felt in various parts of the body, including the joints, kidneys and intestine.

Anaemia
The red blood cells in the child with sickle cell anaemia have a shorter life span than those of a normal red blood cell. This, coupled with the fact that the red blood cell is more fragile than usual, causes anaemia and the child may feel breathless, tired and giddy as a result.

Jaundice
The child may become jaundiced at times due to the destruction of red blood cells.

There is no cure for sickle cell disease. The child will probably be admitted to hospital in a crisis, and he or she will need reassurance, pain relief and rest, and fluids should be encouraged. Folic acid supplements may be prescribed. Folic acid is needed for red blood cell formation. Infections will be treated. Sometimes a blood transfusion is needed. Remember, carers must be able to recognise warning signs of impending problems and seek medical advice. Warning signs and symptoms include raised temperature, swelling and pain.

A blood test for sickle cell disease or sickle cell trait (where the person is a carrier) will be carried out routinely on all susceptible individuals before an anaesthetic, in pregnancy and if the symptoms are suggestive of sickle cell disease.

SEX-LINKED INHERITANCE

Muscular Dystrophy

Approximately one in 500 males are born in the UK with this disorder. There are a number of variants; of these, Duchenne's is the most common and the most severe and will be considered here.

There may be a history of delayed walking. There is muscle weakness, and the child may have difficulty, for example, in climbing the stairs. He may walk with a wider gait (manner of walking) than previously. The weakness is progressive, and the child may have lost his independence by the age of nine or ten. Ultimately the heart and respiratory muscles are affected. The child usually dies during teenage years as a result of respiratory tract infections due to the extreme weakness.

There is no treatment, and care is aimed at prevention of wasting of muscles by physiotherapy and keeping the child comfortable. Consideration will need to be given to conditions at home, and it may be necessary for an occupational therapist to organise some alterations to assist the care of the child. The child and parents will need specialist counselling to help them to come to terms with a condition that is progressive and ultimately fatal.

Haemophilia

Approximately one in 10,000 males are born with this condition, in which there is a disorder of clotting due to the absence of factor VIII haemophilia or the absence of factor VII (haemophilia B, sometimes referred to as Christmas disease). A blood test for clotting time (which will be prolonged) will confirm the diagnosis.

This is a sex-linked condition where the female is the carrier. An affected male will pass the gene onto his daughters, who will be unaffected by the disease but be carriers of the condition. A female carrier will pass the gene onto some of her sons, who will be affected, and to some of her daughters, who will be carriers. (It is possible for a female to have the condition, but for this to happen, the child would have to have a female carrier mother and a father who is a haemophiliac, so this is very rare.)

An affected child may bruise and bleed more easily when he becomes more mobile and may bleed easily when he cuts his first tooth. The carer will need instructions about specific care. The child should be able to have as normal a childhood as possible, but with the carer trying to avoid harm within reason. Haemophiliac children should wear a Medic-Alert bracelet to alert medical and paramedical staff to the condition in an emergency.

Treatment

Any bleeding will need to be controlled. This may be achieved by the administration of Factor VIII, which may sometimes be given by the parents (they will be taught this procedure by the specialists). If the bleeding is not controlled or if there is a major bleed, the child will need admission to hospital.

Note: in the UK prior to 1985, blood was not screened for the presence of Human Immunodeficiency Virus (HIV). The result was that the virus could be transmitted via a blood transfusion or blood products. Tragically, some children and adults were therefore exposed to the virus and some have progressed on to develop Acquired Immunodeficiency Syndrome (AIDS) (see page 106). Blood and blood products are now heated to kill off the virus before any blood is used, but this does not always happen abroad, especially in some developing countries.

Kleinfelter's Syndrome

Here, there are three sex chromosomes (XXY) and the child is male. Characteristically, these children have very long legs, may have a degree of mental retardation and are often sterile as adults.

Turner's Syndrome

Here, there is a single X pattern (XO) and the child is female. Growth is often slow and stunted and there is a web-neck. Ovaries may be absent.

CHROMOSOMAL ABNORMALITIES

Down's Syndrome

In this condition, there is trisomy of chromosome 21 or translocation (when a small piece of one chromosome becomes attached to another pair and prevents its normal activities). The risk of having a child with Down's syndrome increases in women who are older, and it rises significantly after the age of thirty-five.

Screening

The risk of Down's syndrome can be assessed by a recently introduced blood test called the Triple test (also known as the Barts or Leeds test). If this shows a high risk, an amniocentesis, which is more specific, would be recommended. Diagnosis is made on the appearance of the child and confirmed by a chromosome analysis. The child will characteristically have slanting eyes (upwards and outwards), a flatter facial profile, low ears and a wide bridge to the nose. Heart defects are often present.

Many of these children will have severe learning difficulties, but all of them will need to be assessed for their educational needs. Down's syndrome children tend to be prone to infections, particularly chest infections, and suffer from a higher than average incidence of heart disease.

Other Factors Associated with Congenital Abnormalities

KNOWN FACTORS

Maternal infection can result in:

- adverse placental functioning;
- the foetus being attacked by the organism;
- infection of the foetus as it passes through the birth canal.

If the infection occurs during the early stages of pregnancy (the first trimester), the risks of abnormalities of the foetus are higher. Infection later on in pregnancy can result in growth retardation.

Rubella

If the mother contracts rubella in the first trimester of pregnancy, there is a high risk of congenital abnormality. Organs most commonly affected are the ears, eyes and heart. The baby may be born deaf, blind or mentally retarded with heart malformations and is said to have Congenital Rubella Syndrome.

140

HIV

The Human Immunodeficiency Virus, which is thought to be responsible for causing AIDS, does cross the placental barrier. The child may be born with HIV antibodies, but only some of these babies go on to develop AIDS. See page 106.

Herpes Simplex

This is the virus that causes genital herpes. To protect the baby from the disease, an elective caesarian section will be performed.

Medication

Many drugs taken during pregnancy may have an effect on the unborn foetus; for instance, the incidence of cleft palate is higher if the mother is taking steroids. Ideally, the mother should consult a doctor before taking any medication during pregnancy.

Smoking

This has been shown to have an adverse effect on the foetus. Babies born to mothers who smoke are found to be of lower birth weight and are more prone to chest infections, asthma and glue ear.

Alcohol

Women who drink heavily during pregnancy may give birth to a baby with Foetal-Alcohol Syndrome. These children are generally smaller, may have heart defects, have a smaller brain and may be mentally retarded.

Drug Addiction

Babies born to mothers who are drug addicts are more likely to be premature and of low birth weight. They are often jittery and generally agitated.

Rhesus Incompatibility

This causes Haemolytic Disease of the Newborn. The majority of people in the UK are rhesus positive. (Rhesus is a sub-group of blood type.) A rhesus-negative mother has no antigens to the rhesus factor in her blood. If the father of the baby is rhesus positive, the baby will be rhesus positive, as the rhesus factor is dominant. There will be no adverse effect to the first child, as the blood of the foetus and the mother do not mix.

However, at birth, a few foetal blood cells leak into the maternal circulation. These contain the rhesus factor, which the maternal circulation regards as foreign and therefore attacks and destroys. This is done by the mother producing an antibody to the rhesus factor, called Anti D. This Anti D remains in the maternal circulation. In subsequent pregnancies, these antibodies cross into the foetal circulation and start to destroy the red cells of the foetus where the rhesus factor is found. This will lead to the foetus becoming anaemic. The result of this is that, after birth, there is a large amount of bilirubin (the breakdown product of the destruction of the red blood cells) in the blood. If the bilirubin level rises too high it may affect parts of the brain tissue.

Prevention
This problem can be prevented by identifying all rhesus-negative mothers when they first attend antenatal clinics. Anti D is given by injection after delivery, miscarriage or abortion. This prevents the mother producing her own Anti D. However, the injected Anti D is later recognised by the body as being 'foreign' and is removed from the blood stream. Thus it has prevented the mother making her own antibodies and is itself removed from the body before any subsequent pregnancies. Therefore the next pregnancy is not at threat from rhesus-factor destruction.

UNKNOWN OR MULTIFACTORIAL CAUSES OF CONGENITAL ABNORMALITIES

Talipes

This occurs in approximately one in 1000 children. Talipes is a condition of unknown cause where there is deformity of the foot, which is twisted. The condition is sometimes referred to as clubfoot. There are several forms of talipes. Often surgical correction is required, although in mild cases, physiotherapy may be effective.

Congenital Dislocation of the Hip

This is one of the most common congenital defects and occurs in between one in 500 children and one in 1000. Girls are more commonly affected than boys. The condition is more commonly present in breech babies and it occurs more commonly when there is a family history of the condition. It is present when the head of the femur (thigh bone) does not fit into the unusually shallow acetabulum (the cavity in the hipbone into which the femur fits). The cause is unknown, although it is thought that it may have something to do with the maternal hormone levels or possibly the position of the foetus in the uterus. It is usually identified when the newborn is examined; if not, it is often picked up in the child surveillance clinic. Occasionally, it is only noticed when the child starts to walk, and then the condition is more difficult to treat.

In mild cases, abduction (movement away from the midline) of the hip can be achieved by the baby wearing a double nappy. He or she will not usually need any special care other than the usual changes of nappy. The carer, however, will have double the washing load!

In more severe cases a frog plaster may be needed to keep the hips in abduction. Positioning of the baby/child for feeding and cuddling may take a little ingenuity. When the child is a little older and would usually be using a high chair, some modifications will be needed with safety in mind. He or she will need to be washed carefully, with particular care to the skin immediately under the plaster where rubbing and soreness can occur. There will be an area of plaster cut out so that the child can pass urine and faeces. This area is protected with a waterproof material so that it can be kept clean. However, the carer will need to follow advice on positioning of nappies for the younger child or positioning the older child on the pot or toilet.

It is difficult to get the child into a pushchair or pram with ease and it is particularly difficult to transport the child in an ordinary car seat. The hospital may have some equipment to lend which may be helpful. It is imperative that the carer follows advice on lifting safely.

Older children may need to have traction applied in order to correctly position the hip joint. Some children may need to have surgery for congenital hip dislocation. These children may or may not have been in a hip plaster.

Remember, the hospital will issue specific written instructions for the care of children in plaster casts, and these should be followed carefully.

Cleft Palate and Cleft Lip

The child may be born with a cleft palate and/or a cleft (hare) lip. The condition occurs in approximately one in 1000 live births. A cleft palate is a hole or split in the palate, a cleft lip is a split in the lip.

The cause is multifactorial, although there is an increased chance of having a child with the condition if there is a history of cleft palate in the family. Mothers taking steroids during pregnancy also have an increased risk of having a child with a cleft palate.

Deformities such as these are distressing to the parents and family and they will need reassurance that they can be repaired. The baby may have difficulty in feeding. Specially designed teats may help. If there is a large cleft, it may not be possible to breast or bottle feed the baby, in which case the baby is fed with a spoon. Boiled, cooled water may be given after the feed so that curds of milk don't collect around the cleft.

A cleft palate is generally repaired around the age of one to two years, and a cleft lip is usually closed earlier.

During this first year, a child with a cleft palate will have been referred to many specialists, including:

- the orthodontist: it is necessary to mould the maxilla (the roof of the mouth) into a well-formed arch;
- the audiologist: children with cleft palates may have a hearing loss, which may in part be due to the fact that they tend to have repeated ear infections, as the function of the Eustachian tube (the tube that connects the naso-pharynx with the middle ear) may be impaired;
- the speech therapist: the child will see a speech therapist early on, well before he or she can speak, with the intention of developing good speech patterns;
- the plastic surgeon: he or she will generally co-ordinate the various professionals and then operate on the child at the appropriate time.

Heart Disease

A baby may be born with a malformation of the heart or the blood vessels of the heart. The incidence of congenital heart disease is between eight and ten per 1000 live births. It is a major cause of death in babies in the first year of life.

The cause is unknown; however, if the mother has rubella during the first trimester of pregnancy or if she has drunk large amounts of alcohol during pregnancy, the baby is more likely to have heart disease.

Types of heart disease
Atrial and ventricular septal defects: a 'hole in the heart' between the atria or ventricles. This results in blood shunting from the left side of the heart to the right, which means more blood is being pumped

through the lungs. Many will close spontaneously in the first few years of life; some may require surgical closure.

Patent ductus arteriosus: in intra-uterine life, blood bypasses the lungs via the ductus, which closes at birth. Failure to close results in some of the blood flowing from the aorta to the pulmonary artery, and the work of the left side of the heart is increased. Sometimes the presence of this defect is not known until the child is three or four years old. Treatment involves heart surgery to tie off the ductus.

Coarctation of the aorta: a narrowing of part of the aorta, which causes a partial obstruction, resulting in a high pressure of blood before the narrowing and a lower pressure after the narrowing. The heart therefore has to work harder to overcome the defect. Surgical treatment may be necessary; the age at which this is done will depend on many factors.

Valve stenosis: the aortic, or mitral, valve may be thickened (stenosed) and will therefore be less efficient. A replacement valve may be needed.

Fallots tetralogy: there are four defects:
- thickening of the pulmonary valve;
- ventricular septal defect;
- thickening of the right ventricle;
- positioning of the aorta over both ventricles.

The baby may become cyanosed (blue) during activity, for example crying. As the child grows, he or she learns to keep activities in check so that rest periods can be taken. Treatment of the condition depends on the general condition of the child and the age, and will usually involve surgery.

Transposition of the great vessels: the aorta is situated over the right ventricle (not left), and the pulmonary artery is situated over the left ventricle (not the right).
This condition usually results in death unless surgery can be carried out.

The specific care of children with heart abnormalities will depend on the condition and treatment. The parents should be able to give clear instructions on the care needed. Many of these children should be encouraged to have as normal a lifestyle as possible. Some will require regular medication. If surgery is required, the child will usually be admitted prior to surgery for investigations and preoperative care. The parent(s) are encouraged to stay with the child. When the child is discharged, the parents will be given instructions for care.

Spina Bifida

Spina bifida is the malformation of the spinal arch which protects the spinal cord. It occurs in approximately one in 400 births. The disability will vary. Spina bifida occulta is a very mild form of the defect and no specific care is required. Babies with a meningocoele (a sac containing cerebrospinal fluid apparent over the spine) or a meningomyeloecoele (a sac containing cerebrospinal fluid and nerve tissue apparent over the spine) will need surgery soon after birth so that the sac can be covered and protected from drying and possible infection. Some of the children will be paralysed, with urinary and bowel problems. The professionals involved in caring for the child will give expert advice on the care of the baby.

Screening

Blood is taken at sixteen weeks of pregnancy to detect the levels of alphafoetoprotein (AFP). A high level may indicate the foetus has spina bifida, and the mother will be offered an anomaly ultrasound scan which will give a detailed picture of the unborn baby. The cause is unknown; however, it is familial (tends to run in families). There is some evidence to suggest that folic acid deficiency may be implicated as the cause, and women are advised to take folic acid supplements prior to getting pregnant and for the first twelve weeks of pregnancy.

Cerebral Palsy

This is a defect of the part of the brain that controls movement or posture. This damage may have happened before birth, during birth or soon after birth. There is no specific cause, although a number of factors may be implicated. These include anoxia (lack of oxygen) before, during or after birth. The child will have some degree of weakness affecting one, two or all limbs.

Cerebral palsy may be identified soon after birth, but is more commonly diagnosed sometime in the first year of life, when the child may be slow at meeting the usual milestones.

The affected muscles may be floppy (flaccid) or stiff (spastic). There may be evidence of learning difficulties.

There is no cure for cerebral palsy, but treatment is aimed at maximising the child's motor and intellectual development. Soon after the condition is diagnosed, the child may be assessed in a paediatric assessment centre, where many specialists, including the paediatrician, psychologist, occupational therapist, physiotherapist, audiologist and speech therapist, will assess him or her over a period. Together with the parents, a plan is made to give the child the best chance of achieving his or her potential.

Care of the child

The care the child needs will revolve around the outcome of the assessment. It will probably include regular physiotherapy and speech therapy. Schooling will be considered, as will pre-school education. Some will need to go to special schools.

EPILEPSY

This is a result of a sudden, brief disruption of the normal electrical activity in the brain. It affects between four and six children per 1000. Epilepsy can run in families, may occur as a result of brain injury, either before or during birth, and may be caused by a lack of oxygen, infections or low blood sugar, amongst other things.

Classification of epilepsy can broadly be divided into:

* generalised fits;
* generalised absences;
* focal, or partial, fits.

Generalised Fits (grand mal)

These may occur at any age (although they are uncommon in children less than six months), during the day or at night, many times a day or very infrequently.

They are characterised by various phases that may include:

* aura: this may precede a fit and may be apparent to the child. The type of auras that occur are very diverse and can include such sensations as a taste in the mouth or a funny smell;

147

- tonic: the body stiffens due to muscle contraction, and the child falls to the ground. Contraction of the laryngeal muscles may produce a characteristic cry.
- clonic: uncontrollable jerking of muscles – during this time, the child may be incontinent of urine or faeces and produce excess saliva;
- a period of unconsciousness.

This may be followed by a period of sleep, after which the child may be a little disorientated.

Care of the child during a generalised fit
- Ensure that the area is safe. Do not move the child, except to put him or her in the recovery position (see page 48); stay with the child, loosen any tight clothing, but do not restrain the child. After the fit, make him or her comfortable, give reassurance and allow the child to sleep or rest.
- If the child has been incontinent, he or she will need to be washed and given clean clothes. The child may feel acutely embarrassed by this, and the carer will therefore need to be tactful. An older child may wish to see to him or herself.
- If the child hit him or herself during the fall, this incident will need to be reported to the parent (and person in charge if in playgroup, etc.) and the accident book would need to be filled in. If the carer suspects that the child has suffered any adverse effects as a result of the fit, medical help should be sought.
- If the fit lasts more than five minutes or if the child goes straight on to another fit, a doctor should be called.

Generalised Absences (petit mal)

These attacks occur in approximately two to five per cent of all epileptics. They are characterised by a brief loss of consciousness, and there is usually no muscle involvement. The onset of the problem is usually between the ages of five and nine and frequently ceases at puberty.

The attacks usually start abruptly. The child may drop an object due to a slight loss of muscle tone, but it is uncommon for the child to fall to the ground. The attacks usually last for a very short time – five to ten seconds – and the child will stare blankly ahead often blinking or slightly twitching.

These absences are frequently missed or, if seen, put down to lack of concentration. The child can usually follow on with the activity or conversation he or she was involved with prior to the absence, but may need to be reorientated.

These absences can cause problems with schoolwork if they are frequent, due to the many periods of loss of consciousness. They may also cause problems if the child has an attack whilst swimming or riding a bicycle.

Care of the child during a petit mal fit
- If you suspect a child in your care has petit mal, report your suspicions to the person in charge or to the parent.
- It may be necessary to reorientate a child who has just had an attack, and a gentle reminder should help.
- The child should always be accompanied when swimming, and specific advice may be necessary.

Focal or Partial Fits

These are divided into simple and complex fits. Only part of the brain is affected in this type of epilepsy.

Simple partial fits
Consciousness is not impaired. They are characterised by either a sensation – for example, numbness or tingling – or rhythmic twitching or jerking of a limb (or part of a limb).

Complex partial fits
There may be an aura; the child may then appear distracted or confused and repeat a series of movements which serve no purpose, such as lip smacking or plucking at clothes. Sometimes this type of epilepsy may be difficult to detect.

Care of the child during a focal or partial fit
Ensure that the area is safe and talk to the child; often they can still hear and will find this reassuring.

General Information

Known epileptics are advised to wear a Medic-Alert bracelet. They do not need to go to hospital unless they do not recover from the fit. Medical assistance would be required for any child not previously known to be epileptic. The parent or carer should inform playgroups, nursery school, schools or clubs that the child is epileptic. At the same time, it is helpful if some information about managing the fit could also be given so that any unnecessary fuss can be avoided.

Fits can usually be controlled by using medication. There are various anti-convulsant drugs available, and the specialist will prescribe the one most suited to the child. It is important that the therapy should be taken as directed. If medication is forgotten, there is a possibility of another fit occurring. There is a tendency for children to improve spontaneously.

STUDENT ACTIVITIES

Genetic Inheritance

I   It is likely that you will be involved in caring for a child with a congenital abnormality at some time in your career. You are working in a day nursery as a supervisor. When a new child is due to start at the nursery, the parent(s) provide general information and also information on illnesses and medication. Over the next year you will have a:

- six-month-old child with cystic fibrosis;
- two-year-old with a recently repaired cleft palate;
- four-year-old with sickle cell disease.

Design individual questionnaires that you could give to the parents, asking the questions to enable you to give the best care for the individual children.

Congenital Disclocation of the Hip

I   Prepare a leaflet for parents and carers which gives information on caring for a child with a frog plaster. Include suggestions on modifications of equipment the child would need.

2   Plan activities for a day for the following children in a frog plaster: a six-month-old baby and a two-year-old child.

150

13

HOSPITALISATION

In most hospitals, children are cared for on children's (paediatric) wards where the parent(s) are usually welcome to stay. Visiting times are unrestricted, so that even if the parent(s) cannot stay, they are welcome at any time.

Parent(s) are encouraged to care for the child as much as possible, thus reducing the child's anxiety at what can be a stressful time. Hospitalisation can be distressing. Much of the preparation and care given to young children is aimed at trying to reduce this distress.

Emotional Reaction to Hospitalisation

Psychologist John Bowlby helped to finance research in the 1950s by James and Joyce Robertson on the effects of separation on young children. The Robertsons made a series of films entitled *Young Children in Brief Separation.* These films recorded the behaviour of children in hospital or in residential nurseries. Bowlby and Robertson outlined the three phases of response to separation that may be shown by the child when left in hospital.

Protest
The child will cry and cling to the parent in an attempt to prevent them leaving. He or she will become very distressed when the parent leaves and may cry uncontrollably.

Despair
The child realises that the parent is not going to return. He or she is inconsolable, but eventually appears to settle in. However, he or she is often quiet, uncommunicative and appears sad and may regress. The child becomes upset and angry when visited.

Detachment
The child 'settles down'; he or she accepts the situation and may show indifference to the parent on return. This stage is seen less commonly

than the other stages, but may be reached if the child has been in hospital for a long time and has been cared for by many different carers. He or she will appear to be happy, but is trying to ignore the hurt of losing his or her parents.

Note: it is important that anyone caring for a child who is in hospital or going into hospital is aware of these stages and understands them so that the child can be cared for sensitively.

The effects of these reactions can leave the parent(s) distressed and the child totally bewildered by the whole experience. In the past many children took a long time to overcome the effects of hospitalisation, suffering nightmares and anxiety.

As a result of the work on separation by Bowlby and Robertson, the Platt report (1959) was published to encourage the nurses of sick children to care for their psychological as well as physical needs. One of the recommendations was that provision should be made for mothers of children under five to stay with their child. Later, the voluntary agency National Association for the Welfare of Children in Hospital (now called Action for the Sick Child) was set up to 'raise awareness of the emotional needs of all sick children'. The reaction children show to hospitalisation depends to some extent to their age.

FACTORS THAT MAY AFFECT A CHILD'S REACTION TO HOSPITALISATION

Age and Stage of Development

Birth to six months

A baby will generally have been cared for on a one-to-one basis. He or she will be affected by the changes caused by hospitalisation. The parent(s) are usually encouraged to stay in the hospital with the child and to care for him or her as much as possible to provide security.

Six months to two and a half years

The child between these ages has a relatively limited vocabulary and is not yet able to understand all that is said. He or she will have built up a firm relationship with the parents or carer and is often distressed by separation. Separation anxiety is more apparent at this stage, and the child will often protest loudly. He or she is also affected by changes in routine, and regression is common.

152

It is important that the parent/carer should stay with the child if possible; if it does prove impossible, then he or she should be encouraged to make full use of open visiting.

Pre-school

Separation anxiety is still a feature in this age group and may manifest itself in the child being excessively clingy, refusing to eat, having sleep problems or withdrawing. Many children of this age see illness as some sort of punishment, and if adequate preparation is not given, worries and anxieties are more apparent.

It is recommended that the parent or carer stay with the child. The child has built up a trust in him or her, he or she will be able to offer simple explanations, using language that the child understands. Honesty must be used at all times, because the child will lose trust in the parent/carer if he or she is misled. The pre-school child may fear separation from parents more than the operation.

School age

Most children in this age group are capable of understanding a simple explanation of why they need to be hospitalised, but frequently worry that they are missing something important. It is a good idea if the parent/carer stays with the child, although depending on the nature of the admission and the individual child, it may be acceptable to both if full use is made of unrestricted visiting.

Relationship with Parents

Children who are insecure are likely to find hospitalisation more stressful.

Preparation of Parents

Parents are the best people to prepare children for hospital. They therefore need to be adequately prepared themselves and should be aware of:

- the importance of their presence when the child is in hospital and their role;
- what will happen to the child whilst he or she is in hospital;
- the nature of separation anxiety;
- ways in which the child might react in order to cope with the anxiety;

- the need for kindness and honesty;
- the knowledge that their anxiety may increase the child's anxiety.

The Child's own Knowledge of Hospitals

If the child has been told that if he or she behaves in a certain bad way he or she will be 'taken to the hospital', hospitals may be perceived as places to fear.

The child may have some first-hand experience of hospitals, perhaps through visiting a relative. This experience may be negative or positive, and it may help to discuss 'the time you visited . . . . . . in hospital'; this may provide a forum for the child to express worries.

The initial impression of the hospital is often what will be remembered, and it is therefore important that the carers should strive to make that experience as positive as possible.

Separations from the Family

A child who has some experience of being away from the family for short times may have positive or negative memories of the experience, and these will influence the ability to cope.

PREPARATION FOR ADMISSION TO HOSPITAL

Children will be admitted to hospital either as an emergency or planned admission. The amount of preparation that can be done with a child admitted in an emergency will be limited. However, children who have some preparation are less frightened than those who have none. Rodin (1983) stated that children who are prepared for hospital and medical procedures cope better than those not prepared.

A recent recommendation from the report from the Department of Health on the Welfare of Children and Young People in Hospital (1991) states that:

Children should, (therefore) be admitted to hospital as in-patients only if appropriate care cannot be provided daily in the community.

Whether for in-patients or otherwise, paediatric wards and departments should provide an environment which is conducive to the promotion of health and the lessening of stress, with both emotional and clinical health needs receiving constant attention.

154

Points for Consideration

The child may be:

- frightened of the unknown;
- frightened by stories he or she might have heard about hospitals;
- worried about being away from his or her family (however, parents should be made aware that there are facilities for them to stay with the child and that these may be available at no extra cost);
- worried about how to behave;
- frightened about the loss of his or her independence;
- wary of strangers;
- worried about the food he or she might be expected to eat;
- worried that he or she will be in pain;
- worried that he or she may be left in hospital (particularly relevant if the child is not visited often).

Preparation

Leaflets
Hospitals often send out leaflets or a booklet to the parents to share with the child some weeks before the child is due to be admitted. Although the hospital sends these out early, it is a good idea to delay sharing them with the child until about a week before the child is due to be admitted. The leaflets or booklet will usually contain information about the ward, such as:

- things to bring into hospital;
- mealtimes;
- facilities for parents to stay;
- the role of the parent when the child is in hospital;
- school;
- play and the playroom;
- saying goodbye (even if parents are staying in hospital with the child, they will need at least a short break);
- safety;
- doctors' ward rounds;
- what happens after the child goes home.

Books and toys
Children love to be read to and they will be able to gain information about hospital by listening to books being read. Libraries usually have a good selection of books on the subject of children in hospital. Toys can also be used effectively in the preparation. Fuzzy-felt hospital allows the child to make up hospital scenes and can be used particularly effectively with pre-school children, as can Play Mobile hospital, and, of course, dolls and teddies.

Pre-admission visits
Increasingly, hospitals are offering pre-admission visits for children due to be admitted in the near future. The child, parents and any siblings are invited to come into the hospital to meet members of staff and to see the ward for themselves. They are given a tour of the ward, shown the beds and the lockers, the toilets, the playroom and the toys. They are also shown some of the equipment that is commonly found on a children's ward, such as a stethoscope. The Rogue's Gallery is pointed out to the children and their families (see page 62). These visits are usually arranged for a Saturday as it is usually more convenient for the family. Children often spend some time in the playroom playing with the toys and meeting the play specialist.

Preparation in the child's workplace (playgroup, nursery school and school)
Many experts feel that preparation for hospital should be included in pre-school and school activities, thus allowing the children to gain positive images which will encourage them to talk and play, thereby acting out their worries. It is important that any questions about hospitals should be answered honestly and in language appropriate to the child's understanding.

Preparation the day before admission
Allow the child to be involved in packing the things he or she will need in hospital. The booklet will probably give a list of things the child will need. It will include:

*   a sponge bag (containing a sponge or flannel, a toothbrush and toothpaste, soap, talcum powder (if used), comb or brush);
*   towels;
*   clothes (he or she will probably be dressed for most of the day);
*   night clothes;

- slippers and shoes (some hospitals have an outside play area);
- a few favourite toys, books or tapes (ideally these should be named);
- a comforter if one is used (again, this should be named);
- favourite drink and some non-perishable food (check with the nurse in charge);
- family photographs to put on the bedside table;
- nappies (if appropriate);
- special bottles or feeders;
- the Personal Child Health Record (see page 9);
- books and magazines for the child and the parent(s).

Tell the child what will happen. Use language that he or she will understand. Always tell the truth, and if you don't know something, say so, but promise that you will find out when you arrive. If a parent or carer is going to stay, tell the child – it will reassure him or her that someone familiar will stay. If no one can stay, tell the child how often someone will visit. Answer the child's questions – he or she will often want to know a lot of different things about being in hospital.

The day of admission

It is a good idea to keep the routine as near to normal as possible. If the child is going in for surgery as a day case, the parents may have been told not to give the child anything to eat or drink after a certain time. It is very important to adhere to these instructions, and if the child is old enough to understand, then he or she should be told. However, with a younger child, it may be a case of organising the rest of the family to eat earlier or later than usual, so that the child doesn't see the food.

When the child arrives on the ward, one of the nurses will already be allocated to organise the child's care and will greet him or her. The nurse will introduce him or herself by the first name (this helps keep the situation as informal as possible), talk to the child and thus start to build up a rapport. The child will be shown his or her bed, introduced to other children and told where his or her parent will sleep (if staying). The nurse will then take the parent and child to find some toys to play with whilst the child is formally admitted to the ward. The nurse will then gather information about the child by talking to the child and parent so that an individual care plan can be drawn up.

General information, including name (and any pet name), age, date of birth, next-of-kin (including family unit), siblings, immunisations to date, religion and special cultural practices, will be gathered either before admission or at this stage.

On admission, the parent(s) are asked about the child's past medical history, including any admissions to hospital. They will be asked what they (and the child) understand the reason for admission to be, so that any misunderstandings can be clarified if necessary. Any allergies and medications the child is taking will be noted.

The carer (and child, if appropriate) will then be asked for information on the child's usual routine. The nurse also needs to find out the following specific information.

Communication
A child's ability to communicate will vary according to the age, stage of development and, to some extent, the personality of the child. The nurse will find out what is normal for the individual and if the child requires any communication aids, such as a hearing aid or glasses.

Hygiene
The nurse will need to establish the usual routine, which includes bathing, washing and cleaning teeth.

Rest and sleep
The child's usual pattern of naps and sleep will be noted and will include information on where the child sleeps, the usual sleeping position and any bedtime routines.

Comfort
Many children have comfort habits, and these often become important during stressful situations such as hospitalisation.

Food and drink
The nurse will need to find out if the child is bottle fed, breast fed or weaned. He or she will also need to find out whether an older child can feed him or herself. Any dietary restrictions will be noted.

Play and activity
This will depend on the age and stage of development and includes information on the child's mobility. Any favourite toys or games will be noted.

Elimination

The nurse will need to establish if the child wears nappies, whether he or she is toilet trained, any special words that he or she may use and the child's level of independence. The nurse will also need to find out the child's normal bowel habits.

THE CARE PLAN

Having gathered the information, the nurse, together with the parent(s), will write a care plan for the child. At this stage, the role of the parent will also be discussed, and the nurse will find out if the parent(s) are going to stay with the child.

Note: the older child (aged five or over) will be expected to study each day (providing he or she is considered well enough).

Implementation

The care plan will be put into operation, and changes or alterations will be made as necessary.

Evaluation

The plan is evaluated, and reassessment made as necessary.

Soon after admission, the child will be examined by one of the doctors. He or she will need to examine the child and may request some investigations. These will be explained to the child and the parent(s). Other professionals may now meet the child, depending on the nature of the reason for admission.

THE IMPORTANCE OF PLAY FOR THE SICK CHILD

Play is essential for any child for physical, intellectual, social and emotional development. It allows the child to learn about the world, learn new skills, get on with others and act out fears and fantasies. It remains an essential part of the day, even when the child is unwell. The child may be able to come to terms with the illness more easily if he or she is allowed to play and act out his or her feelings. Play is an ideal medium through which children learn to cope with stress.

The sick child usually regresses and prefers to play with toys that he or she discarded some time ago. These toys require less concentration and are therefore more enjoyable for the child while he or she is unwell.

Specialist play workers are employed in most hospitals and are in overall charge of play in the ward. Most hospitals have a playroom on the children's ward, and the children have access to painting, sand, water, dough and cooking, as well as puzzles and books. There are usually televisions and video recorders on the ward, and they are increasingly equipped with computers. Some hospitals also have some sort of outdoor play facility.

Hospital play can:

- be used to help in the preparation of children for specific procedures;
- allow the child to act out any fears and anxieties;
- take the child's mind off the situation and, since children play as part of their daily routine, help to restore some of the normal aspects of life.

The hospital corner in the playroom can provide the child with the opportunity to act out fears and anxieties. This corner will need the following equipment:

- syringes (no needles);
- bandages;
- masks;
- stethoscopes;
- bed;
- dressing-up clothes;
- dolls and teddies.

The play specialist may be involved in preparing children for the following procedures:

- surgery;
- intravenous infusion;
- change of dressing;
- X-ray;
- physiotherapy;
- removal of sutures.

The specialist will talk the child through the procedure with the aid of photographs and the equipment. The child may be encouraged to try on a mask and then look at him or herself, play with the stethoscope and listen to his or her own heart sounds (easily heard, even through a Fisher Price stethoscope). Other equipment will be made available as necessary.

Play is part of a normal day to the child, so that, by playing, some sort of normality remains in the child's life during this very stressful time.

When providing play facilities, the carer must consider:

- the mobility of the child;
- the age and developmental stage of the child, taking into account regression;
- use of suitable materials; for example, sand is not really suitable for a child wearing a plaster cast;
- that he or she may need to be the partner in a game;
- that a hospital corner is invaluable in a playroom;
- that some children are isolated because of their condition, and the play specialist is a very important visitor who may help to relieve the boredom.

Mobility

The mobile patient can take him or herself to the playroom; the immobile patient can be wheeled to the playroom in a bed. With preparation, the bed can be protected in such a way that the child can paint, use modelling clay and participate in other messy play. Mirrors can be positioned so that reading in bed is easier, and for the patient who cannot turn the pages, a page turner can be attached to the book rest.

Age and Developmental Stage

The sick child will often find that his or her concentration span is shorter than usual, and, as already seen, children do regress when unwell. Toys designed for a younger age group which require less concentration are better.

The Play Specialist in the Intensive Therapy Unit

Children in the Intensive Therapy Unit may be critically ill, but they may still benefit from some sort of play.

The unconscious child will often be able to hear (hearing is the last sense to be affected when a person becomes unconscious), and listening to music or having a favourite book read will be reassuring to the child.

Any carer involved in looking after unconscious children should always remember that many of these children can still hear and that it is always important to tell the child what you are going to do before doing it so that the child is aware of what is happening.

Children who are very unwell but not unconscious will often enjoy looking at mobiles or perhaps a poster placed where he or she can easily see it (this may be on the ceiling). The child can listen to a book being read or to music.

As the child improves, he or she may be ready for more active play sessions. The play specialist may work with the other professionals, for example the physiotherapist, so that activities involve play and thus will be more enjoyable for the child.

It is important to realise that play in such situations should be for short periods, as the child may tire easily after the stimulation.

THE CHILD ADMITTED TO HOSPITAL AS AN EMERGENCY

The child admitted to hospital without some of the preparation discussed above may be more anxious and will therefore need some special attention. The nurses, play specialist and others involved in the child's care should be made aware of the situation and will need to explain everything to the child and his or her parents. However, the same principles of care apply, whether the child is admitted as an emergency or as a planned admission.

PREPARATION FOR RETURNING HOME

When the child is considered ready to be discharged from hospital, a meeting should be set up with the parents so that a suitable time can be arranged. Research has shown that, when people are stressed, they do not retain all that is said to them; instructions about medication and care will therefore need to be written down. They should be given telephone numbers to contact in case they be worried.

Parents will need to be told that some children do display some disturbance after being in hospital. However, this is less of a problem if the parent has stayed in the hospital with the child or if the child has been in hospital for only a short time. The child who does react to the stay in hospital may show signs of one or more of the following.

Regression
The child may want to be cuddled more than usual; may wet him or herself when he or she has previously been dry or may revert to a more babyish way of speaking. This behaviour will usually last for only a short time, and the parent is best encouraged to go along with it. The child needs the parents' time and reassurance.

Aggression
The child is responding to the frustration of being in hospital, and any aggressive behaviour should only last a short time.

Sleep disturbance
Some children may want to sleep in the same room as their parents after being in hospital, because they are anxious after their hospital stay. Some children will have dreams or nightmares, which will gradually lessen as the child gains confidence again.

Problems in school
The child's teacher should be made aware of the possibility that these may occur so that he or she can show understanding.

It is important that parents are made aware of these possible reactions to hospitalisation so that they can respond positively and considerately to the child, knowing that he or she will overcome them.

STUDENT ACTIVITIES

Preparation for Admission to Hospital

1   Prepare a leaflet (no more than two sides of A4 paper) that could be sent out to parents before the pre-admission visit. Include in your leaflet all the information that you think would be beneficial to the parent and enable them to help prepare the child for hospital.

2   When answering a child's questions, honesty is important, as is answering questions in a way that the child will understand. With reference to your knowledge of human growth and development and your specific knowledge of speech and language, how might you go about answering the following questions?

- When the doctor takes my appendix out, can I keep it? (a five-year-old)
- Will it hurt? (tonsillectomy in a three-year-old)

- Why can't I stay here [at home] and have the operation, you could look after me? (a four-year-old)

The Importance of Play for the Sick Child

I   Make a list of activities that you could do with children aged three to four in a playgroup, so that you could introduce them to the idea of hospitals. Ask in one of your work experiences if you could try out one or two of your ideas. How will you evaluate the activity? Discuss the ideas with your tutor.

14

CHILDHOOD CANCERS

—

Many different types of cells make up the body, each of which has a role to play in its smooth running. These cells will multiply at the correct rate for the individual to ensure that:

- growth takes place until such time as the adult size has been reached;
- old or worn-out cells are replaced.

Cell division is usually carefully controlled. However, if continuous and unrestrained cell division occurs, abnormal cells are formed which crowd out normal cells and cause damage.

This over-production of cells results in a growth referred to as the **primary growth**, or **tumour**, and the cells do not function as they should. Some tumours are non-malignant (benign), others are malignant (cancerous). Benign tumours may need to be removed by surgery.

Malignant tumours (cancers) can affect the functioning of cells around them. Some of the malignant cells may break off and spread to another part of the body, usually by the blood stream or by the lymphatic system. These are referred to as **secondary growths** or **metastases**. Metastases can destroy the function of the cells they invade.

Types of Cancer

There are many different types of cancer, just as there are many different types of cells. They are classified according to the cell and tissue type from which they originate.

The most common types of childhood cancers are leukaemias, cancers of the brain and lymphomas.

Causes of Childhood Cancers

The cause of most childhood cancers is unknown. However, there is some evidence that ionising radiation, viruses and genetic factors may play a part in the causation of some cancers.

Unfortunately, since very little is known about the causes of childhood cancers, little can be done to prevent them. However, child carers should keep themselves up to date with information on any research that may identify causes in the future.

Diagnosis

This depends to some extent on the carers of the child being aware that something is not quite as it should be. It may be that the child:

- has been excessively tired;
- appears pale;
- has lost weight;
- has been generally unwell for some time;
- has developed a lump or lumps that may warrant medical evaluation.

Sometimes signs or symptoms may be picked up in the child surveillance clinic.

If cancer is a possible diagnosis, the child is usually referred to a regional centre for that type of childhood cancer.

TREATMENT

At present, there are three main types of therapy that are used in the treatment of cancer. These are:

- surgery;
- chemotherapy;
- radiation.

Surgery

The aim of surgery is to remove the cancer so that the function of the body can be restored and spread prevented. Surgery is most successful for cancers that are limited to an area and have not spread. It may also be used as a palliative (alleviates the symptoms but does not cure the disease) measure when the cancer is causing symptoms that cannot be easily controlled by other means. Surgery may be followed by radiation and/or chemotherapy treatment.

Radiotherapy

Radiotherapy is used in the treatment of cancer to cause the death of cells or a decrease in the growth of abnormal cells. It may be used to shrink the size of the cancer, thus relieving the symptoms, and it can be used as a curative treatment. The dosage of radiotherapy is carefully calculated to minimise damage to surrounding tissue. It is sometimes given after surgery to destroy any remaining cancer cells.

Unwanted side-effects of radiotherapy
The child may be excessively tired after treatment and may feel nauseated or actually vomit. There may be loss of hair from areas that have been treated. Sometimes the skin around the treated area is red and sore. The carer will be given specific instructions on the care of this area.

Chemotherapy

Chemotherapy is the treatment of disease by drugs. There are a number of drugs that can be used to destroy the cancer cells. They do, however, have some effect on normal tissue. They are used particularly in cancers that are widespread, such as leukaemia. Chemotherapy may involve the use of cytotoxic drugs. These work by destroying abnormal cells in the body and are particularly effective against the rapidly dividing cells which include cancer cells. Unfortunately, they may also destroy other rapidly dividing cells, such as those in the gut, the hair and in the bone marrow where blood cells are produced.

167

Unwanted side-effects of chemotherapy
The unwanted side-effects include hair loss, diarrhoea, vomiting and anaemia. The child is also prone to infections, because the cytotoxic therapy can destroy the production of white blood cells in the bone marrow. Antibiotic therapy, either as treatment or prophylactically (as a prevention against infection) may be given.

Leukaemia

Leukaemia is the condition that occurs when the bone marrow produces too many white blood cells, many of which are immature and abnormal and therefore do not function normally. (White blood cells help the body to fight infection. There are different types of white cells with slightly different functions.)

It is the commonest type of cancer seen in children.

TYPES OF LEUKAEMIA

Leukaemia is defined according to:

- the type of white cell affected;
- whether the onset is acute or chronic.

In children, acute leukaemias are more common than chronic leukaemias. Acute leukaemias have a sudden onset, chronic leukaemias have a slower onset and take time to develop.

CAUSE

The cause is unknown; however, there are several factors that may be involved.

Radiation
Children of mothers who received abdominal X-rays during pregnancy have a slightly higher risk of developing leukaemia.

Viruses
Research has shown that leukaemia may be the result of an abnormal response to a viral infection.

Chemicals
Some chemicals may cause leukaemia.

Congenital factors
There is an increased incidence of leukaemia in children with Down's syndrome.

The Effects of Leukaemia on the Child

The child is prone to infections. The over-production of white cells generally results in a preponderance of immature cells. These are incapable of fulfilling their role of fighting infection. The effects of the infections are that the temperature may be raised. The child therefore feels hot and uncomfortable. The appetite is usually suppressed, and the child may lose weight. The body will attempt to respond to the infection, and the lymph glands will swell (see page 33). The child may complain of pain, the nature of which will depend on the origin of the infection, for example, the child may also complain of pain in bones (white blood cells are manufactured in bones), and this is due to the excessive over-production of white blood cells.

The over-production of white blood cells results in other blood cells being under-produced. The child may therefore suffer from anaemia (a condition which arises if there are insufficient red blood cells). A child who is anaemic will be tired, may be breathless (particularly on exertion), pale and generally listless.

The over-production of white blood cells also results in the under-production of platelets (these are needed for blood clotting). The child will therefore bleed more easily, bruising is often noted more frequently than previously and he or she may be prone to nose and gum bleeds.

DIAGNOSIS

This is made after the child has been seen by a doctor, a blood test taken and the increased numbers of white cells and decreased numbers of red cells and platelets noted. The child will go into hospital to have confirmation of the diagnosis made by a bone biopsy (when a small amount of bone marrow is taken and examined).

TREATMENT

The aim of the treatment is to destroy the abnormal cells. This is hopefully achieved by the use of chemotherapy and sometimes radiotherapy. The child will usually need several courses of treatment, and this may be continued for a long time. When a blood test shows no evidence of the immature cells, the child is said to be in remission. However, the treatment is usually continued after this time, because there is a chance of a further relapse.

Sometimes a bone marrow transplant may be performed when the child is in remission. Bone marrow transplants are only possible if a suitable donor can be found.

The survival rates for children with leukaemia have improved tremendously during recent years, and the five-year survival rate was as high as 70 per cent during the period 1983–1985 for children with acute lymphoblastic leukaemia.

Tumours of the Nervous System

Cancers of the nervous system cause the highest number of cancer deaths in children after leukaemias. They are the commonest type of solid tumour (abnormal cells that are all in one clump). The cancers of the nervous system can arise from various areas in the system, such as the nerve cells, the supporting tissue and sometimes the blood vessels in the nervous system.

Brain Tumours

The effects of a tumour in the brain is related to the space taken up by it. These cancers can be primary or secondary cancers. It is uncommon to see brain cancers in children under the age of two years.

The child will often have a headache, which is characteristically worse in the morning. The effect of the headaches and the general condition of the child may lead to irritability. The growth leads to a rise in the pressure within the skull, which is known as raised intracranial pressure and is responsible for the child feeling nauseated and perhaps vomiting. Other effects of the growth will depend on where it is in the brain: visual defects may occur, such as double vision, squints or nystagamus. Hearing

170

defects may also occur, and there may be muscle weakness. If the growth is pressing on the cerebellum (the part of the brain at the back of the skull), the child may be ataxic (lose full control of body movements), although sometimes growths in this area may lead to the child becoming clumsy, and this can sometimes be overlooked initially. Tumours in the brain can also cause the child to have fits. As the condition progresses, the child may lose its appetite and thereby lose weight.

DIAGNOSIS

The parent or carer will take the child to the doctor, who will examine the child. The doctor may find evidence of raised intracranial pressure and other relevant symptoms. The child will then be sent to the regional unit, where he or she will be investigated further. Investigations include a skull X-ray, a CAT (computerised axial tomography) scan, and perhaps magnetic imaging. An EEG (electroencephalogram) may be requested to see if the electrical impulses across the brain have been affected.

TREATMENT

This will depend on the nature and site of the growth. It may be possible for the neurosurgeon to remove the growth completely if it is well defined and in an accessible place. In some cases, radiotherapy may be used to shrink the growth, and this is used particularly if the growth is invasive and inaccessible for removal. The effectiveness of treatment depends on many variables: the size, accessibility and type of growth and whether or not it has invaded other structures. There may be complete recovery, some disability or, in some cases, the treatment may be unsuccessful.

Other Tumours in the Central Nervous System

The nervous system is made up of the brain, the spinal cord and the peripheral nerves. Tumours in the spinal cord are less common than those in the brain, and may be impossible to remove. Growths may arise from the peripheral nerves, but generally these are benign. Sometimes the cancer from one area in the body will metastasise to the spinal cord, and this is usually inoperable.

Tumours of the Urinary Tract

The most common cancer of the urinary tract is a Wilm's tumour, also known as a nephroblastoma. The cause is unknown. There is an increased incidence among siblings and identical twins, which suggests a genetic tendency.

THE EFFECTS OF WILM'S TUMOUR

The carer may notice or feel a swelling in the child's abdomen, commonly at bathtime. It may also be picked up when the child is being routinely examined for an illness. Some children may pass blood in their urine. There may be other general symptoms of malignancy, such as weight loss.

DIAGNOSIS

Abdominal X-rays will reveal a growth, and other investigations will then be carried out to confirm the diagnosis. Tests are also carried out to ascertain the presence or otherwise of metastases.

TREATMENT

The child will have the growth surgically removed, either completely or as much as possible. This is followed by radiotherapy and chemotherapy. The survival rates for children with Wilm's tumours are the highest of all the childhood cancers.

Lymphomas

These are solid growths that arise in the lymphoid tissue, mainly the lymph nodes and the spleen. They are subdivided into Hodgkin's lymphomas and non-Hodgkin's lymphomas.

EFFECTS

The child will have enlarged lymph glands. He or she may have a raised temperature and night sweats (when the child sweats excessively at night, so much so that he or she may wake and will need to be washed

172

and have a change of clothing) may be a problem. The child will be more prone to infections than usual and may be anaemic. Nausea and vomiting may also be a problem.

DIAGNOSIS

Several tests may be carried out, including taking a biopsy of the lymph gland. Blood is taken and examined, X-rays and scans are carried out, so that an accurate assessment can be made of how advanced the illness is.

TREATMENT

This usually involves radiotherapy and chemotherapy. Generally, Hodgkin's disease can be treated successfully in childhood.

Bone Cancers

Bone cancers are uncommon in children.

EFFECTS OF BONE CANCER

The child will complain of pain over the affected site. There may be evidence of a lump, which is painful.

DIAGNOSIS

This is usually confirmed by X-rays and scans.

TREATMENT

This may include surgery to amputate the affected limb and chemotherapy.

Skin Cancer

Children rarely develop skin cancer, but the carer needs to be aware of the measures needed to prevent its development in later adult life.

ROLE OF THE CARER IN THE PREVENTION OF SKIN CANCER

• Keep children out of the sun when it is at its most intense (between 11.30 a.m. and 2.30 p.m.), ideally longer. Carers should therefore plan the day around these times.

173

- The child should be dressed in a cotton dress or T-shirt (ideally one with a collar), shorts and a floppy hat.
- Sunscreens (factor 15 or above) should be worn whenever the child is exposed to the sun. They should be reapplied after swimming.
- If children need to be outside when the sun is intense, they should make use of the shade.

Caring For Children with Cancer

(Here it is presupposed that the child's parents have been involved in the care and management of the child during the treatment and the early stages.)

The long-term outlook for children with cancer has improved over the last decade. It is important for the child to maintain his or her normal routine as much as possible, so that he or she can enjoy the same activities as before becoming unwell.

PRE-SCHOOL AND SCHOOL ACTIVITIES

The child will obviously be absent for periods because of the illness or the treatment, either at home or in hospital. Liaison between the family and teachers or carers is essential so that the child can return with the minimum fuss. Teachers or carers will usually keep the class in touch with an ill pupil so that he or she does not feel left out. Sometimes it is necessary to ask the parents if an explanation can be given to the rest of the class so that the other children have some understanding of the situation. It is important to give any information in simple terms, so that the other children understand. This is particularly important if the child's physical appearance has changed – for example hair loss – so that the child is not teased by other children.

During the acute phase when the child is in hospital, the teachers in the hospital liaise with the child's own teacher, so that the child can follow on when he or she is feeling up to work.

On returning to school or pre-school activities, it is important that the teachers and carers are aware that chicken-pox or measles can be very severe illnesses in children with cancer and that if any of the other children or adult is unwell with either of these conditions, it must be reported to the parents of the child as soon as possible. The child can then be taken to the doctor or the hospital and given an injection which will provide temporary immunity.

The child's family will have been through a traumatic time and they might appear to be over-anxious and protective. The teacher or carer needs to be supportive during this time. It might be helpful if the teacher or carer writes to one of the voluntary agencies or gets in touch with a self-help group, so that he or she can improve understanding and thus be in a better position to give support.

CARING FOR THE CHILD AND FAMILY AFTER DIAGNOSIS

The effect of a child being diagnosed as having cancer can be devastating to a family. It affects the whole family (parents siblings and extended family).

A senior doctor will tell the parents the diagnosis. He or she will explain about the disease, its effects on the child, the treatment available and the expected prognosis. An explanation of the nature and course of the disease after treatment is given, so that the parent(s) understand the terms 'remission' (improvement in the symptoms of the disease) and 'relapse' (return of symptoms). Experience will allow the doctor to judge just how much information to give at one time.

The child will need care and support because of the illness. The family, health care workers and often voluntary organisations all have a role to play in this. A social worker may be appointed to support the family and to liaise between the hospital staff and the family. The family will be given a phone number as a contact point for questions and they are often given the number of the self-help group. Leaflets and books are also made available.

The parents will need to tell other people involved in the child's life of the diagnosis, so that they are aware of the situation. They will need to be ready to support the child when he or she returns from hospital. Parents need to be aware of the effect a very ill child may have on the lives of siblings who will need time to discuss worries and anxieties as perceived by the other children. They may have feelings of guilt because of arguments and disagreements they have had in the past. They may be affected by the long periods of absence when their brother or sister is in

175

hospital. This may lead to a succession of carers looking after them, which in turn may result in them feeling left out.

THE EFFECT ON THE CHILD

The child's understanding of the illness will depend on several factors including his or her age, developmental stage and the effect of the illness.

The child may have to go through a lot of traumas during the stages of diagnosis and treatment. Much of this time may be spent as an in-patient in hospital, which in itself can be a traumatic experience (see chapter 13). The treatment may have unwanted side-effects, some of which will make the child feel wretched, for example vomiting, or may affect the child's appearance, for example hair loss. The individual care plan must take into account the effect of the treatment and include information on how to help the child cope with unwanted side-effects. The child may also be affected emotionally; unwanted effects of treatment can lead to fear and anxiety about further treatment, long-term hospitalisation will decrease contact with friends and family. An older child may worry about relapses.

STUDENT ACTIVITY

You are working in a reception class as a classroom assistant. A five-year-old child has recently been admitted to hospital for treatment of leukaemia. The teacher has discussed with you the idea of writing to the child, with each child in the class contributing. You are aware that their written skills are limited. Draw a spider diagram to give an overview of how you might plan the session. Consider what you will tell the class members about the child in hospital (this would need to be considered with the child's parents, the class teacher and yourself), what activities each member might be able to contribute, and your role in the activity.

15

TERMINAL ILLNESS AND CARE

—

A child is said to have a terminal illness when he or she is unwell, when treatment no longer has any prospect of curing the disease and death will ultimately result.

The medical team involved will offer help and support to prepare the parents for the eventual death. The aim is for the child to die with dignity. At all times, a very high standard of care is given to make the child as comfortable and happy as possible. The place of death will depend to a large extent on the wishes of the family and the child, and this may be at home, in a hospice or in hospital.

A child may die:

- as a result of a congenital abnormality that is incompatible with life;
- unexpectedly, for example as a result of cot death;
- suddenly, for example as the result of an accident in the home or a road traffic accident;
- as a result of an acute illness, such as meningitis;
- as a result of a prolonged illness, for example cancer.

Caring for a Child in Hospital

A child may die in hospital if he or she is too ill to go home. The parents and sometimes siblings will be offered accommodation either on the ward or nearby.

The parents will be encouraged to be with their child during the last weeks or days. They will be able to give the child much of his or her daily care, with the professionals giving treatment as necessary. The parents will be able to take breaks at any time, and help and support will be offered.

Caring for the Child at Home

Parents will sometimes request that the child be brought home to be cared for by them. This will be discussed with the doctors, and if it is felt possible, the parents will be given every support from the doctor and other members of the Primary Health Care team. Facilities are available for pain or symptom relief to be given. In some areas, there may be a children's hospice which will offer respite care.

Caring for the Child in a Hospice

A hospice provides care for the terminally ill and children with life-threatening illnesses which may not be imminently terminal. The hospice may be attached to a hospital. The care offered is personalised care, and more attention than usual can be given to each child. The hospice will often provide respite care, which is essential because parents can become exhausted providing twenty-four-hour care for the child.

Wherever the child is cared for, parents and carers are encouraged to allow siblings and other children close to a dying child to help in his or her care. Siblings are usually aware that something is wrong, and it is often better to involve them in doing something positive so that they feel that they helped in some way.

Parents and carers should be honest with children and tell them the situation in language that they understand. They should be allowed to express their thoughts and feelings with the adult, who should accept their reaction (which may be unexpected). However, questions will often come later. Comfort should be natural; children can comfort adults as well as adults comforting children.

Bereavement

If at all possible, the parents will be called to be with the child if it is thought that death is imminent. Unless the child dies unexpectedly, the parents will have been prepared to some extent. However, prepared or not, the moment of death usually comes as a great shock.

178

After death has occurred, the parents should be allowed to stay with the child and to hold and talk to him or her and to each other. This should not be hurried. Later, they may wish to help lay the child out.

GRIEF

Adults and children may go through various stages of grief: some individuals react immediately and some reactions are delayed.

Initially, there may be denial and shock, as the bereaved have not yet accepted the fact of death. The funeral is the opportunity for people to say final goodbyes, and this may enable the family to start accepting that death has occurred. Feelings may be a mixture of anger, guilt, anxiety and depression. Siblings may be clingy during this phase. The grieving phase may be thought as being over when the situation has been accepted without extremes of feelings.

SUPPORT AFTER A CHILD HAS DIED

The family doctor will usually visit the family on several occasions to offer support and counselling. The Health Visitor may also visit several times. Sometimes, the children's ward or the hospice offer self-help support groups for parents and/or siblings. If there are any problems associated with siblings or parents coming to terms with the death, the family may be referred to specialist counsellors.

COT DEATH (SUDDEN INFANT DEATH SYNDROME – SIDS)

'Cot death' is the term applied to the sudden unexplained and unexpected death of an infant. Most cot deaths occur between the ages of twenty-eight days and one year and it occurs in approximately one per 500 infants; the cause is unknown. However, as a result of epidemiological studies, various risk factors have been identified:

- the sleeping position of the baby (there is a higher incidence of cot death in babies who sleep on their fronts);
- the temperature of the room (the baby should not be allowed to get too warm);

- cigarette smoke (infants who are exposed to cigarette smoke before and after birth are at higher risk);
- method of feeding (breast feeding has been suggested as having a lower risk for cot death, however the evidence is inconsistent).

It is more common in winter, and boys are affected more often than girls. It is more common in:

- babies born to parents in lower social classes;
- babies born to young mothers;
- babies who have lots of siblings;
- premature babies;
- babies of low birth weight;
- babies of multiple births.

Prevention

Sleeping position

Babies should be put down to sleep on their back or sides. There is no evidence to suggest that they might vomit and inhale in this position. (See figure 28.)

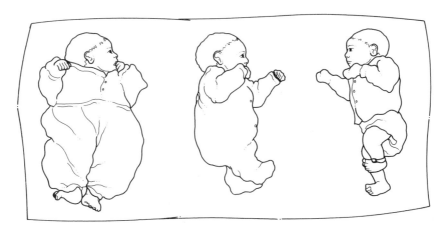

Figure 28   Safe sleeping positions for babies   Babies should be laid down to sleep on their backs or on their sides, with the lower arm forward to stop them rolling over.

There are some exceptions, and these will be advised by the doctor (they include babies with gastro-oesophageal reflux (backward flow of stomach contents) and others with specific airway obstructions).

Smoking
A baby should not be exposed to cigarette smoke, either before of after birth. The risk increases with the number of cigarettes smoked.

Temperature
Overheating is associated with cot death and therefore needs to be avoided. An infant is at increased risk of cot death if he or she is too warm, particularly if the infant has a raised temperature. The carer can check the temperature of the baby by placing a hand on the baby's abdomen, which should feel neither too hot nor too cold.

Other Factors Implicated as Risk Factors

The Foundation for the Study of Infant Deaths has suggested that infants should sleep in the same room as their parents until six months of age, and that they should be in a cot by the side of the parental bed, but not in the parental bed.

Breast feeding should be encouraged wherever possible. It has many benefits and few disadvantages, although the evidence from published studies does not consistently show that breast feeding affects the risk of cot death.

Parents, and others who are entrusted with the care of infants, should be encouraged to seek medical advice promptly if an infant is unwell or thought to be unwell.

Recommended guidance to parents and others who have responsibility for the care of infants (taken from the Report of the Chief Medical Officer's Expert Group on the Sleeping Position of Infants and Cot Deaths).

- The room where an infant sleeps should be at a temperature which is comfortable for lightly clothed adults, i.e. 16–20°C.
- When indoors, infants need little more bedding than adults.
- Bedding should not be excessive for the temperature of the room.
- Bedding should be arranged so that the infant is unlikely to slip underneath; for example, it can be made up so that the infant's feet come down to the end of the cot.
- Duvets should not be used for an infant under the age of one year.

- Bedding should not be increased when the infant is unwell or feverish.
- An infant should not be exposed to direct heating whilst asleep, for example from a hot-water bottle, electric blanket radiant heater.
- An infant over one month, at home, does not need to be kept as warm as in the hospital baby nursery.
- An infant over one month of age should not wear hats indoors for sleeping, unless the room is very cold.
- When infants are taken outdoors in cold weather they chill rapidly, and it is essential that they are adequately wrapped.

If a Cot Death Occurs

The parent or carer who has found the baby may start artificial resuscitation. An ambulance and doctor should be called. The doctor will certify that a cot death has occurred.

Support for the Parents and Carers after a Cot Death has Occurred

The parents will be told that a post-mortem will be necessary and that if the cause of death cannot be explained, it will be registered as a sudden infant death (a post-mortem is carried out on any child or adult who dies unexpectedly).

The parents should be allowed to say goodbye to the child. They should be allowed to hold him or her and be given privacy during this time.

The coroner will arrange for an inquest, and the parents may be asked to identify the child. The police will require statements from the parents; this is the usual procedure for any unexpected death. Once the death is registered, the funeral arrangements will be made. The doctor and health visitor will help and support the family during this time. The mother may need advice on the suppression of lactation. The parents will probably want to talk and ask questions. They will require time from various professionals. The siblings must also be considered, as they too will grieve for the baby (see page 178).

Parents should be told about 'normal grief' and its pattern. There are several self-help groups that they may be put in touch with. The role of the carer must not be forgotten; although not necessarily a relative, the carer may be very close to the infant, especially if he or she is the nanny.

The health visitor will call and often provide a sympathetic ear. Sometimes the parents may need extra help and support with other children.

STUDENT ACTIVITY

Cot Death

I   You are working in a day nursery. Although you are not in charge, you take part in the induction of nursery nurse students for their work experience. You have been asked to prepare a teaching session lasting for twenty minutes on the safety of sleeping babies.

You will need to allow time to find out what the students already know about the subject. How will you go about finding out? (Perhaps you will ask questions and respond to answers? Perhaps you will prepare some written questions requiring short answers?)

You will need to cover the most important aspects of safety in this session, but will need to build on the information in subsequent sessions. What information do you think you will need to feed back to your supervisor?

183

Conclusion

Research continues to expand knowledge and develop new treatments. Just as health professionals must keep abreast with important new changes in their profession to ensure that all children benefit from modern advances, so you too, as the carer, need to keep up to date in child care. Information may be accessed from magazines, books, leaflets (available, for example, in libraries and doctors' surgeries), television and radio programmes. Courses are often run in local colleges or through social services, and you should make an attempt to attend those relevant to your work.

A knowledge of local support groups will come in useful; for instance, there may be a support group for parents and children with special needs. There are many voluntary organisations that provide information and support on a wide range of childhood illnesses. The local library will have access to this information.

You should always familiarise yourself with policies in the workplace, particularly those relevant to ill children (for instance, some workplaces have rules regarding administration of medication).

When working with children, there may be times when you are concerned about your performance. It will be mutually supportive if you share such concerns with a colleague or colleagues working in similar circumstances. Confidentiality will obviously be a prerequisite of any such discussions.

You know the child well and can detect slight changes that may suggest illness. The child will turn to you for comfort if the parent is not present. You will be far better equipped to cope with the situation if you have knowledge and understanding of the illness. The child in turn will feel more secure if he or she is in the hands of a confident and competent carer. I do hope this book has provided the knowledge to make you and the child feel secure.

GLOSSARY

——

Amino-acid   The end-product of protein digestion.

Anomaly   Any organ or structure which is abnormal with reference to form, structure or position; a malformation.

Aorta   The artery that leaves the heart.

Appendix   A blind-ended tube leading from the large intestine.

Ataxic   Loss of power governing movements, usually with reference to walking.

Auroscope   An instrument used to examine the middle ear.

Bilirubin   The breakdown product of red blood cells.

Cardiac sphincter   The muscular tissue that is found where the oesophagus meets the stomach.

Cataract   An opacity of the lens of the eye which prevents light reaching the back of the eye.

Cerebro-spinal fluid   Fluid bathing the brain and spinal cord, found also in the ventricles of the brain.

Cytotoxic medication   A medication that damages cells and is used in the treatment of cancer.

Diphtheria   A bacterial infection in the throat, in which a grey membrane may form over the tonsils causing a blockage. The bacteria produce toxins, which may affect the heart and nerves. Rarely seen in Britain these days because of the effective immunisation programme.

Ductus arteriosus   The blood vessel that connects the pulmonary artery and the aorta in the foetus; the blood thus by-passes the lungs. It usually closes at or soon after birth.

Enzyme   Substance that accelerates the breakdown of food for absorption.

Exacerbation   A worsening of the condition as demonstrated by the signs and symptoms.

Femoral pulses   A pulse that is felt in the groin. Both femoral pulses should be of similar strength.

Five-year survival rate   The percentage of people living five years after the diagnosis of a specific cancer.

Fore-milk   The milk that is contained in the ducts of the breast; it is less rich than the hind milk (which is only released by the let down) which contains more nutrients.

Histology   The study of the structure of tissues.

Hydrocephalus   An excess of cerebro-spinal fluid around the brain, resulting in the child having a large head.

Incubation period   The time between being infected and the appearance of signs and symptoms.

Invasive   The destruction of healthy tissue by a malignant tumour.

Ketones   Breakdown product of fat metabolism.

Neurosurgeon   A surgeon who specialises in surgery to the brain and nerves.

Nucleus   The central part of a cell.

Nystagmus   Fine, jerky movements of the eyes which are involuntary.

Ophthalmoscope   An instrument used to examine the back of the eye.

Poliomyelitis (polio)   A viral infection affecting the nervous system. Rarely seen in Britain today because of the effective immunisation programme.

Prognosis   The probable result of a disease.

Pyloric sphincter   The muscular tissue that controls the passage of the stomach contents into the small intestine (duodenum).

Remission   Lessening of the effects of the disease and possibly the temporary disappearance of the signs and symptoms.

Retinoblastoma   A rare tumour of the retina.

Ribrecession   When the muscles between the ribs are sucked in (may be seen in severe asthma).

Salivary glands   These are situated near the mouth and secrete saliva. They include the parotid gland, the sublingual gland and the submaxillary gland.

Space blanket   A foil blanket designed to prevent further heat loss when used as per instructions.

Tetanus (lockjaw)   A bacterial infection in which the muscles of the jaw and neck go into spasm. Uncommonly seen in Britain because of the effective immunisation programme.

Toddler   A child aged between one and two and a half years.

Tonsillectomy   Removal of the tonsils.

Trimester   The first third (of pregnancy).

Vernix   The waxy substance that protects the skin of newborn babies.

Vesicles   Small, fluid-filled blisters.

BIBLIOGRAPHY

—

Barnes, A. *Personal and Community Health*, Balliere Tindall, London, 1987.

Bee, H. *The Developing Child*, HarperCollins, London, 1992.

Black Report – Inequalities in Health, Penguin, Harmondsworth, 1984.

BMA *Complete Family Encyclopaedia* Dorling Kindersley, London, 1990.

DHSS *Prevention and health: everybody's business* HMSO, London, 1976.

DHSS *Present Day Practice in Infant Feeding: third Report*, HMSO, London, 1988.

DOH *Immunisation against Infectious Disease*, HMSO, London, 1992.

DOH *The Children Act 1989*, HMSO, London, 1989.

DOH *The Sleeping Position of Infants and Cot Death*, HMSO, London, 1993.

Felscher, H. (ed.) *Stedman's Pocket Medical Dictionary*, Williams and Wilkins, London, 1993.

Furley, A. *A Bad Start in Life – Children, Health and Housing*, Shelter, London, 1989.

Hall, D.M.B. 'Health for all children: a programme for child health surveillance'. The report of the Joint Working Party on child health surveillance. Oxford University Press, 1991.

Hilton, T. *The Great Ormond Street Book of Baby and Child Care*, The Bodley Head, London, 1991.

Levene, S. *Play it Safe*, BBC Books, London, 1992.

Lewer, H., Robertson, L. *Care of the Child*, Macmillan, London, 1983.

Morton, J. and Macfarlane, A. *Child Health and Surveillance*, Blackwell Scientific Publications, Oxford, 1991.

Parker, M. and Stucke, V. *Microbiology for Nurses*, Balliere Tindall, London, 1987.

Robertson, J. and J. *Young Children in Brief Separation: a guide to the film series*, The Robertson Centre, London, 1976.

Rodin, J. *Will This Hurt?*, R.C.N., London, 1983.

Sacharin, R.M. *Principles of Paediatric Nursing*, Churchill Livingstone, Edinburgh, 1986.

Sheridan, M. *From Birth to Five*, first published by Nfer 1973, second edition by NFER-Nelson 1975, now published by Routledge, London, 1992.

Stoppard, M. *Baby and Child Health Care Handbook*, Dorling Kindersley, London, 1991.

Weller and Barlow *Paediatric Nursing*, Balliere Tindall, London, 1991.

Weller, B. *Helping Sick Children Play*, Balliere Tindall, London, 1980.

Whaley and Wong *Nursing Care of Infants and Children*, Mosby, St. Louis, USA, 1983.

Wolfe, L. *Safe and Sound*, Hodder and Stoughton, London, 1993.

INDEX

─

A

abdomen, examination of 36
accident book 117
accidents 115, 117, 118
acetabulum 143
acquired immunodeficiency syndrome
    (AIDS) 106, 139
Action for the sick child 152
alcohol 141
allergens 121
allergy 121
alphafoetoprotein test 146
amino acid 185
anaemia 169
anaesthetist 64
anomaly 185
antenatal care 2
Anti-D 142
anti-histamines 125
antibiotics 3
anus 13
aorta 185
appendicitis 105
appendix 185
aspirin 47
asthma 75, 76, 121
ataxia 171, 185
athlete's foot 111
atmospheric effects 5
atrial septal defect 144
aura 147
auroscope 185

B

bacteria 81
barrier nursing 94
BCG 24, 101

behaviour 26
bereavement 178
bilirubin 185
birth marks 12
Black Report 2, 5
blood sugar level 128
body fluids 108
bone biopsy 169
bone cancer 173
bone marrow transplant 173
Bowlby 151
brain tumours 170
breathing difficulties 74, 99, 100
Bricanyl (terbutaline) 123
bronchiolitis 99
bronchitis 99
bronchodilators 123
bronchospasm 121
bruises 12, 28, 169

C

calamine lotion 89
cardiac sphincter 185
care plan 159
Caring for the child with cancer 174
cataract 15, 185
centile chart 68
cerebral palsy 76, 146
cerebro-spinal fluid 28, 185
chemotherapy 167
chest, examination of 35
chest infections 99
chicken-pox 89
child abuse 77
child and family psychiatric service
    65
choking 118